BREATHING POISON

Smoking, Pollution and the Haze

ANTHONY REBUCK

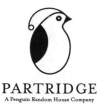

PARTRIDGE

A Penguin Random House Company

Library of Congress Control Number:		2014907215
ISBN:	Hardcover	978-1-4828-9808-8
	Softcover	978-1-4828-9807-1
	eBook	978-1-4828-9809-5

To order additional copies of this book, contact
Toll Free 800 101 2657 (Singapore)
Toll Free 1 800 81 7340 (Malaysia)
orders.singapore@partridgepublishing.com

www.partridgepublishing.com/singapore

Contents

וַיִּפַּח בְּאַפָּיו נִשְׁמַת חַיִּים וַיְהִי הָאָדָם לְנֶפֶשׁ חַיָּה

And He breathed into his nostrils the soul of life, and man became a living soul.[1]

---

[1] Genesis: chapter 2, verse 7

With many thanks for their help, guidance and input to:

Mark E. Cooper
and
Michael S. Rabieh

INTRODUCTION

On May 18, 1980, south-western Washington State and north-western Oregon State in the USA were showered with volcanic ash as Mount St. Helens violently erupted. By world standards, there had been many worse eruptions: Santa Maria in Guatemala, Krakatoa in Indonesia and Mount Katmai in Alaska, for example. Nevertheless, Mount St. Helens was a big one, estimated to be comparable with the serial detonation of 27,000 atom bombs at a rate of one per second for nine hours. An article in the prestigious journal *Scientific American* described Mount St. Helens as having released energy equivalent to 100 times the generating capacity of all U.S. power stations.

The 42 people who died in the vicinity of the terrible eruption asphyxiated from inhalation of volcanic ash. The ash mixed with mucus in their lungs and completely plugged their upper airways. Two people staggered away from the mountain and subsequently died in hospital from purulent tracheabronchitis attributable to inhalation of volcanic ash, hot volcanic gases and particulate matter. Naturally, considerable concern was expressed as to the long-term health and respiratory effects of the disaster.

From the scientific and medical perspective, the response was immediate and thorough. An epidemiological team from the U.S. Centres for Disease Control (CDC) arrived immediately and teamed up with the Washington State Department of Social and Health Services to evaluate the potential health effects. Twenty-seven hospitals in the area were surveyed for their statistics on emergency room visits and admissions for respiratory illnesses. Professor Sonia Buist, one of the most respected pulmonary physicians in the world, happened to be practicing in the region, and she lent her energy and expertise to arranging a conference among all the investigators in 1982 entitled: "Are Volcanoes Hazardous to Your Health? What Have We Learned from Mount St. Helens?"

We have learned a great deal, but in terms of long-term effects, the somewhat surprising finding was that the likelihood of permanent lung damage from silicosis was found to be extremely remote. Exposures were neither high nor long enough to cause long-term harm in the general population; in particular, there was no increased risk of Chronic Obstructive Lung Disease (COPD).

The Mount St. Helens episode indicated that it is not sudden environmental disasters that most endanger human breathing but, rather, more mundane, omnipresent threats that rarely grab the headlines. These omnipresent threats, that is to say smoking and pollution, are responsible for the fact that COPD has risen from seventh leading cause of death and disability in the world in 1996 to fifth at the present time, and predicted by the World Health Organization to be in third place by the year 2020. Tens of millions of people are suffering from moderate to severe COPD with at least three million people dying of it every year. Literally, hundreds of millions of people in the world are suffering from at least the early form of a disease caused solely by the air they breathe.

The disease is treatable and preventable, but remains incurable. For too long the impact of COPD has been underestimated, poorly understood and misdiagnosed.

The growing health care concern regarding death and disability from COPD will affect Asia more than anywhere else in the world. The air has become poisoned in many places by cigarette smoking, automobile and industrial pollution and the haze from illegal wildfires on the Indonesian island of Sumatra. Smoking is the main factor responsible for the development of COPD. The number of smokers is the highest in the world in the Western Pacific Region and China, and continues to rise there, the increase of COPD within Asia will undoubtedly be dramatic.

It is hoped that this book will be a small contribution to public awareness and educational initiatives about the risk of COPD.

CHAPTER 1

Breathing Poison

The advice given by public health officials at the time of the Mount St. Helens eruption was reasoned and appropriate, though not based on scientific evidence because little or none was available at the time. There was no published literature on the effect of volcanic ash on health in May 1980, although such evidence quickly accumulated after the event. People were advised to minimize exposure to ash by staying indoors whenever possible, and to use masks approved by the National Institute of Occupational Safety and Health when outside in the ash. In addition to this sage advice—which is still appropriate in today's battle against smoke haze—the public was told that deposition of ash in the lungs could be minimized by nose breathing.

There is a lot to recommend nose breathing. Indeed, much has been written on the topic, all the way from the second chapter in the first book of the Bible: *"He breathed the breath of life into the man's nostrils."* The nose warms, moistens and filters air before it reaches the lungs and, by being our only sensor of smell, can warn of noxious odorous gases that we might otherwise be in danger of inhaling. The olfactory nerve, or cranial nerve number one, is derived from an embryonic structure known as nasal neural placode. The nerve is so important that it is capable of regeneration if damaged and is the only nerve in the body whose receptor neurons are exposed to the environment, lying bare in the nasal mucosa. Among its other unique features are that it is the shortest of all the twelve cranial nerves and, other than the optic nerve, is the only one that does not join the brain stem but travels directly into the brain. The pseudo-stratified columnar epithelium, otherwise known as the respiratory epithelium of the nose, together with cilia and mucus along the inside wall of the nasal cavity, were ideally "designed" to trap and remove dust from the Mount St. Helens air, which, by any standard, was laden with particles. The particles would have moved down the nasal cavity to the pharynx, where they would have been swallowed or spat out.

The earliest reports of the content of the ash suggested that it contained 60 per cent free silica, enough to lead respiratory disease specialists, present company included, to predict publicly a resulting epidemic of silicosis and tuberculosis. We were wrong, as it turned out, as were the initial reports of the content of the ash. In the initial period of limited information, fears were also expressed about the carcinogenic (cancer-causing) properties of the ash, and there was speculation as to whether it contained radon gas. Eventually, accurate information emerged. The ash particles were on the whole less than 10 micrometres (μm) in size, small enough to penetrate the length of the airways, right down to the alveoli—or air sacks—of the lungs. The good news was that the free silica content of the ash contained approximately 6 per cent free silica, not 60 per cent as originally reported in the media, and of the 6 per cent, 2 per cent was quartz and 4 per cent, cristobalite.

Any long-term damage from the volcanic dust would depend on the composition of the ash, how much was inhaled, the size of the particulates that were inhaled, and the presence or absence of pre-existing lung disease. The exposure to crystalline silica at 6 per cent content, with concentrations ranging from 0.8 to 1.25 mg/m^3, as it turned out, was unlikely to cause silicosis. For the most part, except for the rescue workers on the mountain itself, the general population received only limited exposure, due mainly to the air-cleansing effects of rain, weathering, and the ash becoming worked into the topsoil. Those who were heavily exposed in the first few days experience irritation and inflammation of the upper and lower respiratory tracts, and exacerbation of asthma in those with hyperactive airways. Aside from irritated eyes and a variety of psychological symptoms related to stress, it appears likely that to the extent anyone suffered long-term respiratory consequences, those consequences were quite limited, primarily because the ash deposits were rather modest.

In Asia, the combination of toxic haze from fires, unacceptably high levels of pollution, and pervasive smoking gravely threatens the pulmonary health of tens of millions of people: in sharp contrast to Mount St. Helens, the disabilities resulting from these threats are likely to be permanent and in many cases fatal. As Emerita Professor Sonia Buist and colleagues from Oregon stated (Am J Public Health. 1986), after studying more than 9,000 people over the age of 40 from twelve different countries, "Chronic Obstructive Pulmonary Disease (COPD) is the cumulative response of the lungs to the burden of all that is breathed over a lifetime." Let us consider what it is that people in Asia are breathing today, and the devastating effect it is going to have on their health and well-being.

HAZE

By contrast with the paucity of knowledge that was available about the health effects of volcanic ash before the Mount St. Helens eruption, a great deal of information about haze has been published and was available long before the shocking South-east Asian haze of 2013.

Haze is biomass smoke that arises as a consequence of forest fires and the burning of other vegetation (whether living or dead) and of particles previously deposited on leaves during land-clearing activities. The immediate effect of burning is the release into the atmosphere of gases and particulates, dominated by submicron-size (0.05-0.9 μm) particles that scatter incoming solar radiation and thereby reduce atmospheric visibility and alter regional climate. Since a major outbreak of haze in 1997, Singaporeans have known that acidic aerosols and gases in haze are associated with increased hospital admissions for asthma and other respiratory ailments. Compared with the 2013 haze, the hazes of the 1990s were relatively mild. In 1997, the Pollutant Standards Index (PSI) peaked at a record level of 226. At midday on Friday June 21, 2013, however, Singapore experienced a PSI of 401; a level described in Singapore government guidelines as "life-threatening to ill and elderly persons." Across the Strait of Malacca, just up-wind of Singapore in Sumatra, the PSI reached a shocking 900.

The PSI tells only part of the story, however. Haze contains a complex mixture of particles as well as acidic gases, and Southeast Asia has been experiencing haze from man-made activities with increasing frequency since 1960, with particularly severe episodes occurring in 1990, 1991, 1994, 1997 and 1998. In 1990, haze caused peninsular Malaysia to suffer reduced visibility in the middle of August for at least two weeks. The haze of 1991 was even worse; the region experienced both a volcanic eruption from Mount Pinatubo and a biomass burning that persisted through most of September and October. In 1994, smoke affected 3 million square kilometres in Malaysia, Singapore and Indonesia. Concentrations of sulphur, potassium, titanium, vanadium, manganese, nickel, arsenic and lead in the air were six times higher than average during the haze period in October.

The rest of the world sat up and took notice of the haze of 1997. First, it lasted from May until November. Second, it impacted Malaysia, Singapore, Thailand and the Philippines, not to mention the sources in Sumatra and Kalimantan, Indonesia. The smoke plume reached an altitude of 4 km and included high concentrations of ozone, mono-nitrogen oxides and carbon monoxide.

In 1998, the haze problem was exacerbated by El Nino, which caused an abnormally short wet season and thus reduced the air-cleansing effects of rain. Brunei and Borneo in particular suffered from the beginning of February until the end of April. The PSI levels were as high as 420, and 8-hour guidelines for carbon monoxide levels were frequently exceeded.

Uncontrolled burning from "slash and burn" land clearing in Indonesia caused the Southeast Asia haze phenomenon of 2013. The haze affected several countries as far away as Thailand, the Philippines and even South Korea. The toxic smoke was, as one would expect, at its worst in high-pollution areas such as ports, oil refineries and dense urban areas. Once lit, fires can burn for months and release gases that produce sulphuric acid. In 2013, satellites detected more than 9,000 "hot spots" in Sumatra, with a further 168 in Sarawak. The hot spots were owned by palm oil companies or smallholder farmers who supply palm oil to the large companies and use slash-and-burn methods to clear their land for the next planting season. The president of Indonesia issued a formal apology to Singapore and Malaysia for the hazardous smog, and 2,800 military personnel as well as helicopters and aircraft were deployed to fight the fires.

In Singapore schools and businesses were closed, driving was almost impossible because of poor visibility, and medical consultations for asthma, lung and eye problems increased by 20 per cent. The government issued a warning that the smoky haze "may be life threatening" to vulnerable people. It advised Singaporeans to stay indoors and limit unnecessary activity. Newspaper articles warned of cardiac arrhythmias and heart attacks in people over forty. Many retail suppliers of masks in Singapore sold out of them despite a statement from the British Lung Foundation that "the use of masks is not recommended" since "they are often ineffective and may make breathing more difficult" and a public warning from a British expert that the masks may be sufficient to keep out some particles but not gases that would go straight through them. Dr Keith Prouse of the British Lung Foundation proved to be correct in his prediction that, with respect to, "the concentration of the current smog means it will probably affect everyone in some way." The question that remains unanswered at this time is whether there will be any long-term, permanent damage to Singaporeans' lungs.

In Brunei, Singapore's neighbour on the island of Borneo, PSI levels reached a much more "moderate" reading of 98, but citizens were advised to check the levels regularly and to seek immediate treatment in their nearest hospital if they developed symptoms due to haze.

Smoke had its greatest impact on parts of Indonesia, the source of the forest fires that caused the haze in the first place. Local residents in Riau had to flee their homes; almost a third of them experienced respiratory problems. The haze prevented planes taking off at Syarif Kasim airport as the PSI reached a choking, hazardous level of 900. Twenty-three Indonesian farmers were arrested for lighting fires that started the blazes and a further six for illegal slashing-and-burning. Unfortunately, only small amounts of rain fell during the worst days of the haze, so Indonesia initiated a program of cloud seeding and water bombing. Even when the fires were finally extinguished, they still raged underground in the peat-land, presumably continuing to exude toxic fumes.

Peninsular Malaysia's haze in early 2013 was the country's worst since 2005, with Johor, just across the causeway from Singapore, reporting a PSI of 383, a level described officially as *Very Unhealthy*; 21% of locals reported upper respiratory tract ailments. Much worse was to come. On June 23, Johor experienced a PSI of 746 at 7 a.m., resulting in the declaration of an emergency. The town was in a state of virtual shutdown. Two deaths were reported in one day, one of the unfortunate people being a lady with asthma. Six hundred schools were closed in

Johor alone; sporting events were cancelled, and a warning was issued that those convicted of burning offences would be fined RM 500,000, or imprisoned for up to five years, or both. All schools were closed in Kuala Lumpur, Selangor and Malacca. Pizzas could not be delivered because of concerns about delivery drivers' safety. The choking, vile fumes from the haze were such that for the first time in history, inspection of the honour guard and the opening ceremony of the Parliament session in Kuala Lumpur had to be conducted indoors.

The inhalation of biomass gases in the developing countries of Asia also includes indoor air where wood is used for cooking and heating. Particulate levels in the region of 1000-2000 micrograms $(\mu g)/m^3$ are found where women and children spend many hours cooking over unvented indoor stoves. Studies have shown that exposure to biomass combustion products such as these are a major risk factor for acute respiratory infections, and a leading cause of infant mortality in developing countries. Women who are exposed to biomass fumes as they cook in unventilated areas have been shown to be at risk for chronic respiratory diseases, as well as adverse pregnancy outcomes. The concentrations and duration of their exposure to fumes are far higher than might occur as a result of short-term exposure to biomass air pollution resulting from forest fires. There are serious consequences of exposure to high levels of indoor biomass pollution that include acute respiratory illnesses in children and the development of chronic lung disease in adults. The consequences of indoor biomass pollution are even worse in areas that experience haze from forest fires and slash-and-burn land clearing.

AIR POLLUTION

Many studies have shown, and it is widely believed, that air pollution affects human health. Now for the first time, it has been proven by rigorous research that it also shortens life expectancy.

The research is summarized in a paper recently published in the *Proceedings of the National Academy of Sciences* by Michael Greenstone, a professor of environmental economics at the Massachusetts Institute of Technology (MIT), along with two Israeli and two Chinese co-authors. According to Professor Greenstone, in heavily polluted areas in northern China, where air particulate concentrations were 55% higher than in southern China, life expectancy was 5.5 years lower, on average, across all age ranges. The differences in life expectancy were entirely due to cardio-respiratory causes that had previously not been linked to air quality. The World Health Organization now estimates that 1.34 million premature deaths a year are caused by outdoor air pollution.

With these seminal findings collected from 90 Chinese cities, and with media attention around the world frequently focused on pollution in Beijing, one might think that the worst air pollution in the world was in China. This is not so.

Traffic in Beijing

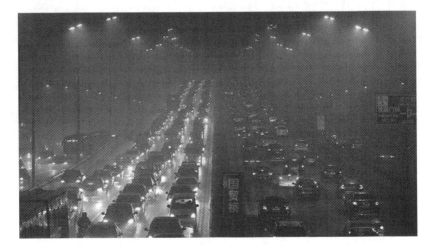

According to the World Economic Forum in Davos, the worst air pollution in the world is in India, followed by Bangladesh and Nepal.

The director general of Nepal's Department of Hydrology and Meteorology, Keshav Prasad Sharma, has said that the fog and pollution in his country simply did not exist ten years ago. It is caused, he says, by burning of wood and cow-dung cake as well as by smoke from industries and vehicles, mainly during the winter. Iqbal Habib of the Bangladesh Environment Movement (BAPA) reports that at times, air quality is so poor that all means of transport come to a complete halt because of zero visibility and work hours fall to as low as four hours a day. The air pollution problems in Bangladesh arise from vehicles, factories, power plants and dust from gravel roads. The pollution is becoming worse year by year, and children and elderly people are increasingly suffering from chronic lung disease. All the while, the number of smoke-belching unauthorized brick kilns is fast increasing. As for India, its Internal Energy Agency says that pollutants and aerosols in the air enhance condensation of water in the atmosphere, causing dense smog. The blankets of smog block sunlight and reduce temperatures. As the temperatures fall, people make more fires from wood, cow-dung cake and hay to keep warm, thereby increasing the pollution. The worst problems according to climate scientists occur during the winter, when the smog cannot escape to the upper atmosphere, forced as it is by cold air blowing in from the northeast that traps pollutants close to the earth.

The World Health Organization lists airborne particles smaller than 10 micrometres—the so-called PM10s—for approximately 1000 cities. The PM10s in these cities comprise mainly sulphur dioxide and nitrogen dioxide from power plants, auto exhausts and industry. An upper limit of 20 micrograms per cubic meter for PM10s is recommended. Above this level, serious respiratory problems in humans occur.

Central Asia suffers the most from PM10s. The world record is held by Ahvaz in Iran, with an annual average of 372 micrograms per cubic meter. The Mongolian capital, Ulan Bator, has an annual average PM10 density of 279, which is only slightly above the levels of Quetta in Pakistan and Kanpur in India. Such cities have made little, if any, progress in improving air quality. For example, the city of Karachi, Pakistan, has attempted to reduce air pollution by replacing smoky buses with vehicles using natural gas, but this small measure is overmatched by increases in smoke both from newly constructed industries and factories and from the burning of more low-quality fuel to produce the electricity to power them.

In India the government has banned the construction of new power plants within the city limits of New Delhi, Mumbai and Kolkata. Existing power plants are being shut down or relocated. Has this turned the pollution tide? Unfortunately, it has not. India's economic boom has led to a huge increase in privately owned cars and SUVs. This is hardly surprising, especially in light of the fact that public transport can best be described as inadequate and the government subsidizes the cost of diesel fuel.

Let us return to China, the focus of MIT Professor Greenstone's recent paper. While Beijing might not be the most polluted city in the world, according to the World Bank report of 2007, 16 of the world's most polluted cities are in China. The health statistics from the World Bank are so disturbing that some official opinions within the country have warned against publishing health statistics lest they produce "social unrest." Nonetheless, the Chinese Ministry of Health now acknowledges that industrial pollution has made cancer the leading cause of death in China and that lead poisoning continues to kill many children. Huge sections of the seas near China are devoid of marine life because of unpleasant algal blooms. Acid rain containing sulphur dioxide and nitrogen dioxide, according to the Journal of Geophysical Research, has spread from China to Seoul and Tokyo and even, it is claimed, Los Angeles.

Noting the rise in China of lung cancer and cardiovascular disease, the president of the China Medical Association, Zhong Nanshan, has warned of the health threats that air pollution, especially from motor vehicles, poses, over and above the harm that smoking causes. Among other things, Dr Nanshan points out that lung cancer is almost three times more common in Chinese cities than in rural areas, despite similar rates of tobacco smoking. The Chinese government has recently stated that air pollution in China is decreasing, but it should be noted that the analyses at the time this statement was made did not include ozone or small particles such as PM2.5 (i.e. particulate matter less than 2.5 micrometres), recorded by some researchers as being in excess of 755µg per cubic meter. How much the concentration of this particulate matter exceeded this level is unknown, since this level represents the upper limit of what can be measured reliably using state-of-the-art technology. These small particles are not reported by the government but are recognized by such international experts as the award-winning environmental journalist Jonathan Watts as being highly detrimental to human health.

Chinese authorities have asked foreign experts to stop publishing "inaccurate and unlawful data," especially when the US Embassy claimed that the air contained 199 micrograms of particulate matter per cubic meter at a time when the Beijing Municipal Council's analysis showed a more modest level between 51-79 micrograms. As for where the truth lies in this dispute, it suffices to say that in 2013, Beijing had average levels of over 300 micrograms per cubic meter, with some recording stations reporting levels of around 700 and even 755 (the upper limit of reliable measurement).

China is planning an inventory of persistent organic pollutants, with the objective of eliminating the production, import and use of pesticides and PCBs. The Chinese are also a signatory to the Stockholm Convention treaty, which seeks to eliminate poly-brominated diphenyl ethers, notorious for their unwanted endocrine effects on humans.

Asia has the dubious distinction of being more polluted than anywhere else in the world. The least polluted cities in the world are Whitehorse, in the Yukon Territory of Canada, and Santa Fe, New Mexico, which have yearly averages of 3-6 micrograms of PM10s per cubic meter. These cities benefit from lower population densities and favourable climates. They are spared the huge influx of former herders and farmers who are pouring into such places as Ulan Bator in Mongolia and who rely on burning coal, wood and dried dung to keep warm and cook meals. Governments throughout Asia, though, are attempting to ameliorate pollution by, for example, enforcing laws regulating manufacturing plant and car emissions. Perhaps most encouraging is the growing public awareness that much of pollution control is in their citizens' own hands. They are becoming more aware of the importance of selecting fuel-efficient vehicles, driving smarter, replacing air filters as they wear out, keeping tires properly inflated, and minimizing vehicular use. Throughout Asia, moreover, we are starting to recognize the importance of "reuse and recycle," of conserving energy, and of substituting renewable energy for fossil fuels. We are also starting to see the growth of facilities for properly disposing of toxic waste.

Unfortunately from a pollution perspective, however, the demand for economic growth is overwhelming efforts to control pollution. In Asia, economic growth is achieved by physical capital expansion and increased energy consumption, with an emphasis on manufacturing and heavy industry. There is no end in sight for this growth, which will likely continue to be based on production in energy-inefficient, polluting industries. Thus, the rewards of economic growth will be tempered by serious threats to human health and well being, not the least of which will be the suffering, disability and mortality caused by Chronic Obstructive Pulmonary Disease.

SMOKING

Abdominal aortic aneurysms most commonly occur in males over the age of 60 who smoke or have smoked. Albert Einstein, whose name is synonymous with "genius", died of a ruptured aortic aneurysm at the age of 76, having undergone surgery for the same condition seven years earlier. Although he favoured pipes—"I believe that pipe smoking contributes to a somewhat calm and objective judgment in all human affairs"—he was not one to turn down a cigar or even a cigarette.

It is only in recent years that smoking has come to be viewed in a negative light. Ancient civilizations, as long ago as 5,000 BCE, smoked incense, originally as part of religious ceremonies, and later cannabis, fish offal, and dried snakeskins for pleasure in social settings and at other times for hallucinatory experiences. In Ayurvedic medicine, "drinking smoke" has been practiced for thousands of years, and in Muslim society, smoking was an essential part of important traditions such as weddings and funerals. We should, however, credit Murad IV, sultan of the Ottoman Empire in the 17th century, for being one of the first rulers to try to ban smoking in the old world. Murad claimed, presciently, that smoking was a threat to public morality and health. Other anti-smoking campaigners, such as the Chinese Emperor Chongzhen, called smoking a heinous crime, and in the Edo period in Japan, growing tobacco was considered to be a threat to the economy by misuse of valuable land that could otherwise be used to plant food crops. Throughout history, however, attempts to ban smoking have failed notwithstanding the fact that they were often enforced with threats of punishment. In 1734 in Moscow, for example, men and women who smoked were threatened with having their nostrils slit. King James 1 in 1604, determined to put an end to smoking in England, imposed a four thousand per cent tax on tobacco, and that failed to stamp out smoking, too. By the mid-17th century, smoking had become part of the culture of every major civilization in the world. Indeed, the notorious Opium Wars were fought over Chinese attempts to ban smoking of the drug, which attempts Britain punished by seizing five of China's ports.

The relationship between smoking and lung cancer was recognized with firm statistical evidence as early as 1929 (by

Fritz Lickint in *Der Tabakgegner*), yet condemnation of smoking was received with little short of disdain for many years. Even Adolf Hitler's Nazi Party preached that women who smoked were unsuitable to be wives and mothers in a German family, and Hitler (Y.S.), for good measure, condemned smoking as a waste of money. That failed, too. By the end of the war, the United States was shipping free tobacco to Germany, and under the Marshall Plan, up to 60,000 tons of tobacco were being shipped to Germany each year and Germans were consuming over fifteen hundred cigarettes each per capita every year.

Although spectacular post-war increases in lung cancer rates occurred in both the US and UK, the numbers were attributed to better reporting and diagnosis rather than an actual increase in lung cancer. Having observed lung cancer death rates in men increasing from 1.5% of all cancers in 1920 to 19.7% in 1947, Richard Doll in 1950 published his seminal work showing the previously unproven link between smoking and lung cancer. His observations were swiftly confirmed by the British Doctors' Study and, in 1964, by the United States Surgeon General's report on smoking and health. Since the report, rates of smoking in the US have halved, and at present, the rate is around 20%. Ironically, though, the number of cigarettes each smoker in the US smokes actually increased in the decade or so following the Surgeon General's report from an average of 22 a day to 30. Throughout the industrialized world, smoking rates have generally declined, but not in China, Laos and Indonesia, all of which are, of course, in Asia; they rank only slightly behind Russia and Greece as the top consumers of tobacco per capita in the world today.

Asia is bucking the smoking trends we are observing in the rest of the world. In the most populous nations in the world, China and India, an increasing number of people are starting to smoke. According to the George Institute of Global Health, the Asia/Pacific region is home to 30% of the world's smokers. According to an article by Prabhat Jha and colleagues in the *American Journal of Public Health*, East Asian countries account for a disproportionately high percentage of the world's smokers (38%). East Asia and the Pacific account for 429 million smokers. The World Health Organization (WHO) has calculated that if people in Asia continue to smoke at the current rate, smoking-related lung cancer rates will double over the next twenty years.

Edouard Tursan D'Espaingnet of the WHO tobacco control program says that in many Asian countries where men already smoke at a high rate, the tobacco industry is targeting women and even children. In China, Indonesia and Malaysia, less than five per cent of women smoke, compared with approximately 60 per cent of men. Women thus represent an a relatively untapped, and therefore enticing, market for tobacco companies, who are using, among other things, fancy cigarette packages such as those shaped like a lipstick stick.

According to reports, at least a quarter of Indonesian children over age 3 have tried cigarettes, and three per cent of them are now regular chain smokers. Smoking is so common among children in Indonesia because cigarettes are cheap and accessible there—costing roughly $1 a pack—and there are virtually no limitations on who can purchase them. The Indonesian landscape is littered with tobacco advertisements that appeal to children on television, radio and in print, from sporting events to music concerts. Another problem is that many Indonesian parents see no problem with their children smoking, and will even give them the money to purchase cigarettes. Some are calling for increased tobacco regulations in the country to curb the child smoking epidemic, but others say that unless parents themselves set an example or, at the very least, restrict their children's smoking habits, the problem of youth smoking will only continue.

In Indonesia, there are 57 million smokers. The Indonesian government recently reported that since 2005, youth smoking rates have doubled. The CEO of Philip Morris International, the largest tobacco company in Indonesia, actually supports stronger regulations and restrictions in Indonesia. The tobacco companies claim, however, that they are not targeting children and are only taking advantage of marketing freedoms that do not exist in other places in order to lure adult smokers from their competitors. For its part, Indonesia's government has promised to cap cigarette output, and it passed a health law in 2009, with some good elements of tobacco control, but the measures have not been enforced as yet. Why? This is presumably because approximately 10% of government revenue comes from tobacco taxes.

Even where smoking in Asia is on the decline, there are troubling signs. In Singapore, for example, smoking numbers have fallen steadily over the last thirty years and are now well below 15%, but there has been a 30% increase in smoking in 18-29 year olds in the last six years and many more minors have started to smoke.

In summary, 700 million Asians smoke every day. Every year approximately half of the world's smoking victims die in Asia as a result of smoking. Cancer and other tobacco-related diseases are rising rapidly.

The secret ingredients in cigarettes.

"Everyone" knows by now that cigarettes contain nicotine, tar and carbon monoxide. Some are also aware that cigarette smoke also contains over 4,000 chemicals, including 43 cancer-causing compounds and at least 400 other toxins.

It is the nicotine that is addictive. After just one puff, the drug reaches the brain in six seconds. It is a very short journey from the alveolar-capillary membranes, into the pulmonary veins, straight into the left atrium—with no intervening valves to slow down the flow—down into the left ventricle and straight into the aorta, pumping at a rate of approximately once per second.

With every puff on a cigarette, a smoker delivers more and more tar to the lungs. The last puff of a completely smoked cigarette contains twice as much tar as the first. Most of the chemicals stay in the lungs, but not carbon monoxide. That particular poison binds to the iron in the haemoglobin in **every** red blood cell in the blood, leaving the red cells unable to carry their full load of oxygen. Carbon monoxide, which is present in all tobacco smoke, has no smell or taste. Smoking one pack of cigarettes can raise the carbon monoxide level in a home to twice the level the Environmental Protection Agency's (EPA) safety limit for **outdoor** air.

There is no secret in the foregoing, as most ingredients of cigarette smoke are well known. There are apparently, however, some secret ingredients, too.

The American state of Massachusetts is trying to compel disclosure of all ingredients by all cigarette makers; its demand has not been warmly welcomed, to say the least, by the tobacco industry. An attorney for the industry has responded by saying that the industry has the right to protect its trade secrets. Some companies have provided lists of ingredients to the federal Department of Health and Human Services, but government officials are not legally allowed to release the information. What is known, according to such prominent physicians, toxicologists and pharmacologists as Lowell Kleinman of California, and K. H. Ginzel of the University of Arkansas is that tobacco smoke contains ammonia, arsenic, benzene, cyanide, lead, formaldehyde and naphthalene (the active ingredient of mothballs). Smokers efficiently extract 90% of particulates and gases in mainstream smoke. Millions of tons of second-hand smoke, i.e., the fumes to which we are exposed in the company of smokers, pollute enclosed spaces, exposing non-smokers to toxins such as acrolein, carbon monoxide and formaldehyde.

Cigarettes, which used to be smoked by role models in theatre, sport and film, are no longer alluring. They are addictive poisons that cause terrible diseases such as cancer and COPD.

The triple threat:

In Asia there is thus a triple threat in the air to human health and well-being. First of all, we are going to see a dramatic increase in tobacco-attributable deaths in low and middle-income countries. Much of this mortality and crippling chronic lung disease can be prevented if smokers stop smoking.

Secondly, there is the threat from air pollution. Additional suffering, disability and premature death from lung disease can be prevented if Asian pollution—the worst in the world—can be reduced.

Last but not least is the threat from haze. The coughing, wheezing and exacerbations of bronchitis caused by the haze—a uniquely Asian problem of smoke from illegal wildfires— would be eliminated if prohibitions against burning were fully enforced.

ACTION PLAN

What can we do about the poisoned environment in which we live?

Smoking

A Cochrane review is an international not-for-profit organisation preparing, maintaining and promoting the accessibility of systematic reviews of the effects of health care. The review found evidence that community interventions using "multiple channels to provide reinforcement, support and norms for not smoking" helped reduced smoking among adults. Specific methods used in the community to encourage smoking cessation include:

1. Implementing policies banning smoking from workplaces and public spaces (comprehensive clean indoor laws can increase smoking cessation rates by 12%-38%)
2. Encouraging citizens to ban smoking from their homes—if you must smoke, smoke outside!
3. Mass media campaigns about the harmful effects of smoking

4. Initiatives to educate the public regarding the harmful effects of second-hand smoke
5. Increasing the price of tobacco products by taxation (it is estimated that an increase in price of 10% will increase smoking cessation rates by 3-5%)

Air pollution

1. Invest time and money in businesses and governments that are working to reduce toxic emissions and improve air quality.
2. Let local government officials know how important air quality is and work with them to find solutions.
3. Improve the quality of life indoors. Do not allow smoking in your home. Choose natural cleaning products. Choose chemicals, paints and glues that are environmentally safe, and keep windows open when using them. Remove debris and dust from home on a regular basis.
4. Use energy-saving methods that reduce the need to burn fossil fuels. Set thermostats so that furnaces and air conditioners are used only when needed. Replace incandescent light bulbs with energy-efficient models. Use a clothesline instead of a dryer.

Haze

1. Strict enforcement of the 1998 ASEAN Agreement on Trans-boundary Haze Pollution (which has not been ratified by Indonesia)
2. Use of financial incentives, the provision of alternatives to burning, and education campaigns to dissuade farmers and developers from slash-and-burn land-clearing
3. Efforts by trans-national organizations such as the Peace Corps to help in local fire-fighting and education efforts

CHAPTER 2

Cough

Chinese Symbol for cough

咳

Dictionary Word of the Day: Chinese cough—*An oriental hack of the throat.*

This is usually sudden and unpleasant. The sound may be harsh and ear piercing. It is comparable to a feline coughing up a hairball.

The ubiquitous cough, cough, cough, hawk and spit that so offend the delicate sensibilities of visiting westerners in cities such as Shanghai, Beijing and Guangzhou, should not. Cough is a partly reflexive, partly voluntary, and physiologically appropriate mechanism for clearing muco-ciliary airways. It is nature's way of clearing breathing passages of secretions, irritants and foreign particles. Frequent coughing may indicate the presence of a disease such as asthma, gastro-oesophageal reflux, lung tumour, heart failure or even the side-effect of a medication such as an ACE inhibitor, but in China, India and the heavily polluted cities of Asia, it is more: it is a protective reflex in otherwise healthy people. The reflex is triggered by stimulation of myelinated afferent nerves as well as non-myelinated C-fibres in the lungs via their rapidly adapting receptors.

According to a recent article in the Journal of Paediatrics, cough is the most common reason for visiting a primary care physician in the United States. The visit stands a good chance, depending on socio-economic status and level of insurance, of initiating the taking of a detailed medical history, sputum culture, and electrocardiogram, as well as X-rays of the chest and sinuses. The objective of good management is to identify and treat the cause, which may sometimes have a psychological component. If no cause is found, based to some extent on the demands of the patient, treatment is likely to be a cough suppressant, expectorant, decongestant, antihistamine, and—if a specialist is consulted—bronchodilators and/or corticosteroids. Should such treatments fail to alleviate the cough, a patient may well put himself or herself in the increasingly popular hands of alternative medical practitioners and try diet supplements, honey, and probiotics such as spirulina, lactobacillus acidophilus, herbal medicine such as peppermint or eucalyptus, as well as homeopathic treatments.

Chronic cough is common in China and is very severe. According to the Journal *Cough*, (www.coughjournal.com) in an article written by investigators from Guangzhou Medical College, over 80% of patients with cough lasting more than eight weeks and having a normal chest X-ray are treated with antibiotics and anti-tussives. The coughing is distressing and anything but trivial; over 50% of women complaining of cough suffered urinary incontinence. Chronic cough in China is increasingly becoming the subject of important research. A common feature among patients is airway inflammation similar to that found in patients with asthma: eosinophils, mast cells and lymphocytes both in sputum and in broncho-alveolar lavage fluid. Microscopy in airway biopsy specimens has shown remodelling, with thickening of basement membranes. Lung washings contain increased levels of inflammatory mediators such as LTC_4, histamine and 8-iso-prostaglandins—all this in non-asthmatic patients complaining only of cough and having normal chest X-rays.

Professor Peter Calverley from Liverpool has shown that patients with chronic cough living in areas of heavy pollution have pathology in their lungs not dissimilar from that arising as a result of passive smoking and the early stages of COPD (i.e., long before the onset of breathlessness). The pathology comprises mucous gland hypertrophy, loss of ciliary structure, and impaired muco-ciliary clearance. Older textbooks would have us believe that cough by itself is of limited consequence in COPD, as though only breathlessness matters as a marker of disease progression. The older texts observed that smoking cessation improved mortality statistics as well as reduced bronchitis symptoms, by which the texts meant sputum and shortness of breath, but cough, taken in isolation, the texts implied, was merely an epiphenomenon, unrelated causally to outcome or progression of disease. This is not correct! Cough has an important influence on well-being, and the majority of patients with COPD complain bitterly about their cough, particularly when it occurs while rising in the morning. As Calverley (2013) points out, patients find cough to be an important symptom, even if their doctors remain to be convinced.

Cough with or without sputum is an early symptom of COPD. It helps to identify people at risk of progressive disease. Smoking cessation early in the natural history of the disease remains the most effective way of reducing cough; non-specific cough suppressants do not work.

In the polluted cities of Asia, even after quitting smoking, there seems to be no escape for most of the inhabitants from inflammation of the airways, the gradual onset of shortness of breath and the inevitable suffering and disability we now associate with COPD.

CHAPTER 3

Asthma

Chinese Symbol for asthma

哮喘

As of the end of 2013, according to the US National Institutes of Health website, there were 3,816 asthma trials being conducted in the world. Children, infants and pediatric patients were the focus of 53.6% of these studies.

An internet search in January 2014, using "asthma" as the search term, yielded more than ten million articles on the subject. Narrowing the search to "asthma treatment" also yielded literally millions of articles. An even more refined search of, for example, "asthma guidelines" still gives more than one and a half million results. All contain essentially the same simple, straightforward advice as to how to reduce asthma symptoms, limit the need for medication, prevent emergency attacks and improve asthma-related quality of life. In summary, the advice is: obtain a written management plan from one's medical caregiver,

take medications as prescribed, keep a diary of symptoms and learn and follow an action plan in the event of an acute attack.
Yet:

1. The prevalence of asthma continues to increase.
2. There is remarkable variation of prevalence rates among different countries.
3. Control of asthma frequently falls short of goals set by current guidelines.
4. The economic burden of asthma is tremendous.
5. Medical treatment is often poor.
6. Many doctors in general practice are unaware of new medical treatments.
7. In some countries, doctors know about new treatments but are, for one reason or another, reluctant to use them.
8. Asthma death rates are increasing, particularly in young people.
9. Nearly all asthma deaths **are preventable**.
10. 250,000 people die of asthma a year.
11. Asthma is under-diagnosed and under-treated.

In other words, although we know how to treat asthma, it is increasing, and more and more people, especially children, are dying from it. Where is this happening? Why? What can be done to reverse the trend?

WHERE ARE ASTHMA DEATHS OCCURING?

Asthma deaths, all of which remain tragic and unnecessary, take place mostly in low—and lower-middle income countries and among lower-income populations. In the US, for example, African Americans have higher rates of asthma emergency room visits, hospitalizations and deaths than Caucasians. For Hispanics, the statistics are even worse: Puerto Ricans suffer asthma at a rate 50% higher than non-Hispanic black people.

The global prevalence of asthma and asthma-related deaths has increased steadily over the past twenty years, particularly in urban areas and especially in Asia. Whereas in Canada and the United States the death rates from asthma are 1.6 and 5.2 per 100,000 respectively, in China 36.7 of every 100,000 asthma patients die.

Singapore, a highly urbanized city-state in Asia, is experiencing 16.1 deaths from asthma per 100,000. The cumulative 12-month prevalence of wheezing in Singaporean pre-school children is now 27.5%. According to the International Study of Asthma and Allergies in Childhood (ISAAC), the prevalence of asthma and allergic rhinitis in other Asian countries such as Thailand has steadily increased since data collection was initiated in 1995. In Japan, during the same period, asthma has doubled, from 4.6 to 9.1%. The trend is similar but even more marked in Taiwan, where childhood asthma has gone from 1.3 to 5.0% during the same period, and the cumulative 12-month prevalence of wheezing and rhinitis in children 10 to 12 years old is now 8.2% and 44.4% respectively. Asthma, wheezing and rhinitis are either rare, or rarely diagnosed in Tibet, but in Bangladesh, 16.1% of the population has asthma, and in Pakistan, the prevalence of asthma and rhinitis has doubled since the start of the ISAAC program. Astonishing statistics are now emerging from Vietnam: 34.9% of children aged 5 to 11 years have allergic rhinitis, and according to Vietnam's Ministry of Health, 48.5% of patients with asthma also have rhinitis.

Across the Asia-Pacific region, according to an Asthma Insights and Reality in Asia-Pacific (AIRIAP) Steering Committee, published in the journal *Respirology*, 27 percent of adults and 37 percent of children reported absences from work or school in one year because of asthma. Among these people, an astonishing 40% required hospitalization, emergency room visits or unscheduled visits to health-care facilities for their asthma in a single year. Vietnam and China reported the greatest number of patients with severe, persistent symptoms. Only 7.5% of people with asthma in South Korea reported missing work because of their disease, but in the Philippines, for reasons that are difficult to explain, the number was an astonishing 46.6%.

Indeed, although Australia is not over-crowded and its citizens enjoy one of the highest standards of living in the world, some disturbing news has emerged recently from that country. The latest Australian Bureau of Statistics data show an increase in asthma-related deaths among children under the age of fifteen years. While overall asthma deaths in Australia continue to decline, for the first time, asthma deaths among children have increased, with 17 children dying from asthma in 2010 compared with 7 in 2006. It is not yet known whether pollution contributed to the deaths, nor whether they occurred in disadvantaged people. Have Australian doctors and their patients become less vigilant, or has childhood asthma become not just more common but also more severe?

WHY ARE ASTHMA DEATHS OCCURING?

Asthma is caused by a combination of genetic and environmental factors and is characterized by recurrent episodes of wheezing, shortness of breath, chest tightness and coughing. The sputum in asthma sufferers is notoriously sticky and difficult to cough up, despite repeated efforts to clear the lungs. This is a marked difference from chronic bronchitis and COPD, in both of which copious sputum is expectorated, particularly on rising in the morning. Characteristically, asthma symptoms are worse at night and in the early morning, or in response to exercise and cold air.

Genetics.

How can genetic factors contribute to an increase in asthma prevalence and severity? The answer probably lies in the phenomenon of epigenetics in which gene activity is inherited without changes in DNA. It is of course well known that family history is a key risk factor for developing asthma in the first place; over 100 genes have been associated, in one way or another, with the condition. These are not "asthma genes" but, rather, play a role in modulating inflammation. The fact, though, that such genes play a role in the development of asthma (where the environmental triggers for asthma are present) does not explain why we are today witnessing an increase in asthma prevalence and severity.

Environment.

The development of asthma, its severity and its exacerbations are greatly affected by the environment—allergens, pollution, environmental chemicals, poor air quality, traffic fumes, etc. The external environment is only part of the problem, though. Inside the home, exposure to dust mites, animal dander, cigarette smoke, cooking fumes and cleaning fluids also increase the risk of developing asthma.

Whether through the mechanism of epigenetics or by directly increasing airway inflammation, changes in the environment are causing an increase in asthma prevalence. As the quality of our environment deteriorates, the frequency and severity of asthma increase. The fact remains, however, that while there is no cure for asthma, symptoms can be improved provided that each patient has a customized treatment and monitoring plan.

Given that the prevalence and to a large extent the severity of asthma are closely related to environmental factors such as pollution, allergens and smoke, can the environment also be blamed for asthma deaths? Probably not, as no less an authority than the Royal College of Physicians has categorically stated that there are preventable factors in 90% of asthma deaths. (While it is uncertain as to why the number of deaths from asthma per year has not fallen significantly, at least in the UK where the death rate has been around 1,200 per year for decades, most would agree that asthma deaths are tragic and unnecessary.)

Over the last decade, age-adjusted mortality statistics in asthma have been re-evaluated employing 21st century population statistics instead of the previously used 1940 population statistics; the newer statistics reflect the generally increased longevity of populations around the world. Accordingly, because most lung diseases increase with age, one would expect death rate calculations to increase under the new standard. Indeed, age-adjusted death rates for asthma are approximately 1.5 times greater when one uses the 2000 instead of the 1940 population. It should be noted, though, that calculations of asthma death rates have been further complicated by revision of the International Classification of Diseases (ICD) coding system used to classify mortality rates from death certificates. When ICD-9 was changed to ICD-10, the calculated death rate from asthma decreased by 11%.

In the 1980s, the death rates from asthma in Australia and New Zealand were, by any standard, high—indeed, among the highest in the world according to published data at that time. In 1989, the standardized mortality rate from asthma reached 5.8 per 100,000 per year in Australia. A number of case-controlled and cohort studies indicated the high death rate was due to preventable factors such as inadequate assessment of severity, discontinuity of medical care, poor adherence to prescribed therapies and inadequate treatment of acute attacks. The Australasian literature specifically mentioned over-use of beta-agonist bronchodilators, and attempts were made to remove at least one of the newer short-acting bronchodilators from the market. A landmark paper in the *New England Journal of Medicine* in 1992 concluded that underuse of preventative anti-inflammatory corticosteroid therapy was more to blame than over-use of any specific beta-agonist.

Are the same arguments regarding asthma deaths still germane today? The answer is not known. The National Review of Asthma Deaths (NRAD), run by a consortium of asthma professional and patient bodies and led by the Royal College of Physicians in the UK, will likely provide the answer. All asthma deaths in the UK are being systematically reviewed and subjected to an in-depth, multidisciplinary, confidential enquiry. We will eventually know the role of the circumstances surrounding each and every death such as medical care received and environmental conditions, so that recommendations can be made regarding how to prevent deaths from asthma in the future.

While the asthma death rates in the UK appear to have remained stable in recent years, asthma mortality seems to be decreasing in the US after a long period of steady increase. The American Lung Association recently issued a report from its Epidemiology and Statistics Unit on trends in asthma mortality and morbidity. The report noted that in 2009, 3,388 people died from asthma in the United States, a figure which represented a 26% decrease over a ten-year period. In New York City, the number of deaths from asthma fell from 213 to 149 over an eight-year period, and the age-adjusted rate fell from 2.7 to 1.7 per 100,000 over the same time.

The overall decrease in asthma mortality, at least in the US, coincided with an increase in the use of inhaled corticosteroids. While it is not possible to prove that inhaled corticosteroids is the sole explanation for the decreased mortality rate, the fact remains that there is a correlation between a significant reduction in asthma mortality and a significant change in asthma management.

WHAT CAN BE DONE ABOUT THE INCREASE IN ASTHMA PREVALENCE AND SEVERITY?

The International Study of Asthma and Allergies in Childhood (ISAAC) reported the prevalence of asthma, rhinitis and eczema in two million children, across 105 countries. (This, incidentally, is currently a Guinness World Record for any collaborative research project on children.) Wading through the 340 articles in over 100 journals that have so far been produced by the ISAAC collaborators is a daunting task, and even now there is not complete agreement as to whether childhood asthma, in particular, is more severe or more common now than it used to be. There is, however, a general acceptance of several important findings:

1. The evidence that genetic factors cause asthma was minor.
2. Most asthma, rhinitis and eczema have a non-allergic basis, especially in developing countries.
3. In developing countries, asthma and allergic diseases are increasing.
4. Prescription practices varied according to socio-economic and ethnic factors.

One can draw a number of conclusions as to the most pressing issues arising from the general literature and, more specifically, the ISAAC data:

First, asthma is under-diagnosed and under-treated, despite excellent management guidelines.

Second, in view of the underwhelming evidence for genetic factors, environmental pollution emerges as a key factor in causing the surge in asthma, particularly in children and most notably in Asia.

TREATMENT GUIDELINES.

The Global Initiative for Asthma (GINA) was born in 1989, the product of a collaboration among the National Heart, Lung and Blood Institutes (NHLBI) and National Institutes of Health (NIH) in the United States and the World Health Organization (WHO).

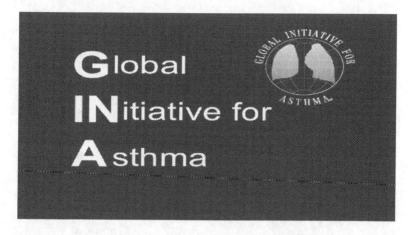

GINA's objectives were to increase awareness of global public health perspectives on asthma, to recommend diagnostic and management strategies, and to identify areas for future investigations. GINA consists of a network of individuals and organizations interested in asthma care who work together to design, implement and evaluate asthma care programs to meet local needs.

Other organizations have also published guidelines. For example, the Malaysian Thoracic Society, the Ministry of Health Malaysia and the Academy of Medicine of Malaysia have published guidelines for management of asthma as a joint statement. The guidelines are extremely thorough and detailed. Indeed, literally hundreds of guidelines for asthma are available, several of which are continuously updated and revised in order to be compliant with new scientific evidence as it becomes available. Among the first asthma guidelines published were those in Australia and New Zealand following the asthma death epidemic of the 1980s. These guidelines had a very significant and successful influence on asthma care in those countries, and they were enthusiastically endorsed and implemented by nurse practitioners. Guidelines such as GINA are evidence-based, and the evidence has changed markedly in recent decades. For example, it was not recognized until the 1980s that asthma results from airways inflammation, which should be treated routinely with inhaled corticosteroids.

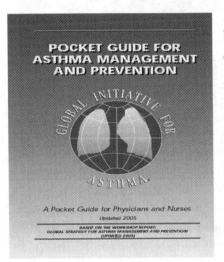

Sadly, there remain gaps between the publication of guidelines and clinical practice, especially in Asia. Investigators from Hong Kong (C.K.W. Lai et al. 2006) have studied the relationship between asthma control and compliance with the GINA guidelines across Asia. As part of the Asthma Insights and Reality in Asia-Pacific (ARIAP) survey they derived Asthma Control Test (ACT) scores in 2,062 patients from China, Hong Kong, Korea, Malaysia, the Philippines and Singapore. They found that only 2.5% of the population met with all the GINA criteria for asthma control in terms of chronic symptoms, nocturnal wheezing, exacerbations and emergency room visits. More than 40% of patients needed urgent care at least once in the preceding 12 months.

Unless guidelines are accepted by opinion leaders, they are unlikely to be disseminated to health care professionals and may well be ignored. Moreover, where there exists a prevailing culture of treatment that conflicts with the recommendations in guidelines. To many physicians in Asia, the concepts in the guidelines are new and appear impractical for use in day-to-day practice. In Asia, traditional medical skills are highly respected, and the guidelines may be in direct conflict with them. Physicians are, however, increasingly being influenced by their well-informed, knowledgeable patients, who get information about their asthma from the internet and confront their physicians with how they believe their asthma should be managed.

Indeed, one of the best ways to improve asthma management in Asia may be to focus on physician education. There is now a growing body of evidence that educational programs for physicians improve asthma outcomes for children of low-income families. A study from the Department of Pediatrics in the University of Michigan has shown that physician education leads to a reduction in the need for hospital and emergency room care in asthmatic children. In Japan, investigators asked why inhaled corticosteroids—a widely recommended treatment in guidelines—are prescribed less frequently than in other developed countries, and they found that the presence of specialists in a treatment facility was the major determining factor as to whether the guidelines were followed.

What can be done to educate and influence physicians to put the guidelines into practice?

Short-term educational programs may improve physician performance. A recent study from Shanghai by Xiao Cong Fang et al. found that among 161 physicians at a training course, only 68% of them actually bothered to attend all of the seven, two-hour sessions. The initial evaluation showed that the physicians did not know the core elements of the guidelines and that their current asthma treatment practice did not comply with guideline recommendations. One might argue that their level of ignorance was due to a scarcity of appropriate medications for their patients of poor socioeconomic status. This rationale does not hold water, as the study was conducted in Shanghai, which has the highest quality of health care in China. The investigators demonstrated an improvement in knowledge of the guidelines during the training curriculum, but the observed effects were small. The investigators concluded that, in order to bring treatment practices into compliance with guidelines, short-term efforts were insufficient; government, regulatory and accreditation bodies must join the fight. Among other things, the investigators strongly support the distribution of easily accessible tools such as algorithms, flowcharts, flow diagrams and pocket guides.

Keeping pace with the guidelines

Well-designed Continuing Medical Education (CME) programs have been shown to have a significant effect on the health status of patients and on health care utilization. The Department of Pediatrics at the University of Michigan has shown conclusively that education provided by local faculty is effective in improving asthma care and in reducing how often asthma symptoms occur and emergency department utilization. An important challenge is to create CME programs that can be widely used by being replicated in new venues with different instructors. Physician Asthma Care Education (PACE) is an interactive physician education program based on underlying theory and sensitive to the needs of primary care providers. The program has been tried in a number of locations in the US and has been shown to retain its effectiveness after a one-year follow-up. Even more encouraging is the fact that the PACE program has lent itself to international travel within the Asia-Pacific region. In Australia, the PACE program was conducted by local physicians and behavioural scientists as facilitators and was sponsored by government agencies. As in the US, the outcomes showed improved physician confidence in developing short-term and long-term care plans, prescribing inhaled corticosteroids, and providing written management instructions to patients. As an added benefit, patient visits with physicians who took the PACE program did not last longer than visits with controls who had not attended the course.

SUMMARY

Asthma is a major global health problem. The disease, particularly in Asia, affects millions of people and places huge burdens on society in the form of medical costs, hospitalizations, drug reimbursement, time lost from work and premature deaths. Many patients have symptoms that affect their quality of life, such as inadequate and interrupted sleep, a reduced ability to exercise and diminished social activities. Many of the deaths from asthma are preventable if asthma is managed properly and patients are educated to act appropriately. It is now recognized that doctors are not adequately equipped or trained with knowledge of asthma management, despite the ready availability of treatment guidelines.

None of this explains why asthma prevalence is increasing everywhere, both in adults and children. The prevalence is increasing chiefly because of poisoned air, particularly in Asia. The poisons we are breathing come chiefly from pollution, smoking and haze, all of which are more severe in Asia than anywhere else in the world—hence, it is vital to reduce these sources of poisons as quickly as possible.

In summary:

1. What is the cause of the global increase in asthma prevalence?
    It is almost certainly environmental pollution.
2. What is the cause of an apparent increase in asthma severity?
    Environmental pollution is the prime suspect.
3. Are asthma death rates increasing in children, having been on the decline for twenty years?
    Suspected but unproven; but if they are, failure to follow treatment guidelines is likely.

CHAPTER 4

COPD:
What Is It, and Why Is It So
Difficult to Understand?

Chinese Symbol for emphysema

肺胀

What is COPD?

Literally: **C**hronic **O**bstructive **P**ulmonary **D**isease.

1. Chronic

A **chronic condition** is a disease that is persistent and long-lasting. The term *chronic* is usually applied when the course of the disease lasts for more than three months. Common chronic diseases include arthritis, asthma, cancer, diabetes and HIV/AIDS. The word chronic comes from the Latin *chronicus*, meaning *time*.

The opposite of chronic is acute.

"Chronic" means constant, not recurrent. A chronic condition never goes away, in contrast to a recurrent disease, which relapses repeatedly, with periods of remission in-between.

2. Obstructive

Obstructive means that the air tubes, or bronchi, are narrowed so that the flow of air in the lungs during breathing is impaired. The person with obstructed airways either has to work harder during every breath just to maintain adequate flow, or the flow of air is simply reduced. The result of having to work harder for every breath is what is known as "shortness of breath" or dyspnea. The result of limited or reduced airflow is an inability to increase breathing during any form of exertion.

Other forms of obstructive lung disease are asthma, obstructive sleep apnoea and bronchiectasis.

3. Pulmonary

Pulmonary means relating to, functioning like, associated with, or carried on by the lungs. Sometimes COPD is referred to as COLD or chronic obstructive lung disease. Both terms mean the same thing. The word pulmonary comes from the Latin *pulmonarius,* meaning *of the lungs.* Doctors who specialize in respiratory or lung disease are sometimes referred to as pulmonologists.

4. Disease

A disease is an abnormal condition affecting our body. It is a medical condition with specific symptoms and signs. Diseases can be caused by external sources, as is the case with infectious diseases, or by an internal cause such as an autoimmune condition.

For our purposes here, disease refers to a condition in which a person suffers from the dysfunction of a major organ system and may also experience distress and social problems.

COPD develops in response to the burden of breathing in harmful matter over a long period. When dust, smoke and poisons are breathed, the airways become inflamed, lung tissue breaks down and the small airways, deep within the lungs, begin to close completely. The first symptom is usually a cough. The cough is typically "productive" of phlegm or discoloured sputum that is either spat out or swallowed. The cough persists and is eventually followed by shortness of breath, at first during exertion and eventually at rest. The course of the disease is inexorable. The symptoms become worse and worse until the unfortunate patient is virtually incapacitated, sitting in a chair, struggling for every breath. Eventually, the strain on the heart, reduction in oxygen, and destruction of blood vessels in the lungs and accumulation of carbon dioxide in the blood can prove fatal.

Although the passage from "smoker's cough" to shortness of breath, heart failure and death are unstoppable, the deterioration is not a steady one. The life sentence of COPD is fraught with acute exacerbations and periods during which the cough becomes more severe, sputum thick and discolored, and shortness of breath more limiting. These acute-on-chronic episodes may respond to antibiotics, physiotherapy, corticosteroids, increased doses of bronchodilators, but recovery is rarely complete. After an acute exacerbation, if the patient survives, his or her health-care provider will notice that lung function has deteriorated below the level recorded before the acute episode, and the patient may admit to a further decrease in exercise tolerance and a reduced ability to take part in and enjoy the activities of daily living.

It will come as no surprise that a life in which one must struggle to breathe, cannot exercise, and has low levels of oxygen in the blood is associated with other co-morbidities, among the most common of which are anxiety and depression. Patients with COPD also have a disproportionately high incidence of coronary artery disease, osteoporosis, high blood pressure and type 2 diabetes.

Anthony Rebuck

What causes COPD?

Smoking tobacco is the primary cause. One can also develop COPD from smoking marijuana and from living in close quarters with smokers, breathing in their second-hand smoke. It is likely that smoking alone causes 80% of COPD. Pulmonologists like to record smoking levels in their patient notes in the form of "pack years," two packs a day for fifteen years, for example, being recorded as 30-pack-years. The effect is cumulative, and the likelihood of developing COPD increases with age and cumulative smoke exposure.

The second most important cause is air pollution. COPD is seen more commonly in people who live in cities than in rural areas, but in the developing countries of Asia, where indoor air pollution from cooking with wood and animal dung is common, so is COPD in women in rural areas.

The third risk factor is occupational exposure, particularly from coal dust, gold mining, textile chemicals such as dyes and cleaning fluids, and fumes from welding. Silica, as we learned from the Mount St. Helens volcanic eruption, does not cause COPD, but it does inflict terrible scarring in the lungs.

Genetics. There is a genetic form of COPD known as alpha-1 antitrypsin deficiency, which is responsible for no more than 2% of cases. In this autosomal recessive disease, a substance called antitrypsin, a protease inhibitor, is missing from our bodies. Antitrypsin protects the lungs from elastase enzymes in white blood cells that escape from neutrophils and break down elastic tissue. Without such protection from antitrypsin, the elastic tissue in the lungs is digested by our own white cells, resulting in a form of COPD known as emphysema. Recent research has now produced a pooled, purified human plasma protein concentrate that can replace the missing enzyme and that can be administered by weekly intravenous infusions, but although the treatment is beneficial, the degree to which the progression of emphysema can be slowed and survival increased is not known.

How does smoking damage the lungs?

Cigarettes, pipes and cigars produce an oxidative stress in the lungs because of the free radicals in the tobacco smoke. The airways in the lung respond to the irritant particles by releasing cytokines. In addition to directly inflaming the airways, smoke impairs the activity of alpha 1-antitrypsin, allowing the enzymes in our white cells to damage our own lungs.

All cigarette smokers who have smoked at least one pack-year have some inflammation in their lungs. Do they all develop COPD? No, but those who do have an enhanced response to the inhaled poisons may develop COPD. The exaggerated or enhanced response begins with the production of excessive mucous, a chronic cough and chronic bronchitis. As the smoking load increases, the small airways deep inside the lungs become inflamed, damaged and disrupted, the condition now having progressed to a stage known as bronch**iol**itis (inflammation of the small bronchi). Finally, as the defence mechanism of alpha-1 antitrypsin is overwhelmed, elastic tissue destruction in the alveoli occurs, and the pathological stage defined as emphysema is reached.

These pathological changes result in increased resistance to airflow in the small conducting airways, large floppy lungs that have lost their elasticity, gas trapping, and progressive airflow obstruction—all characteristic features of COPD.

COPD has become much more common in women, and on the whole, they tend to fare worse than men with the same condition, being more likely to need hospitalization and to die during acute exacerbations. Recent studies have shown that women with COPD have more severe symptoms, greater depression and a worse quality of life than men. They are more susceptible to the effects of smoking and pollution, but fortunately when they quit smoking, lung function improves more than it does in men.

Understanding the physiology of COPD

The end result of chronic bronchitis, bronchiolitis and elastic tissue destruction of the alveoli is that the lungs become big and floppy. A normal lung is like a child's balloon: blow into it, release it, and it deflates all by itself. This is due to elastic recoil of the balloon. By contrast, a COPD lung is like a paper bag: blow into it, let it go, and it just sits there. Like an emphysematous lung, it has no elastic recoil. You cannot empty it unless you squeeze it, just as patients with COPD cannot breathe out unless they voluntarily squeeze their lungs with the muscles of their rib cages and diaphragm.

Patients with COPD have increased lung volume. They look as though they have just inhaled deeply and are holding their breath. Their chest X-ray shows just this: big lungs, heart stretched out vertically, and diaphragms flattened.

Chest X-ray in a patient with COPD.

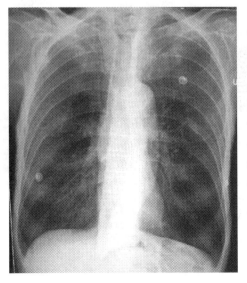

Some people find it difficult to understand why the lungs get big, why the biggest, most expanded parts of the lung are at the top and why the patient cannot deflate his or her lungs and become more comfortable.

This confusion can be removed by turning to the work of two important scientists: Sir Isaac Newton (1643-1727) and Pierre-Simon Laplace (1749-1827).

Formerly, physiologists seem to have ignored the fact that *Homo erectus,* being erect, has erect lungs that, being longer than wide, are subject to the forces of gravity from top to bottom.

In addition, physiologists incorrectly thought that the lung alveoli are equal in size and spherical, as in the classical textbook illustration below. The illustration is incorrect: the alveoli are neither equal in size nor completely spherical. They do NOT look like this illustration!

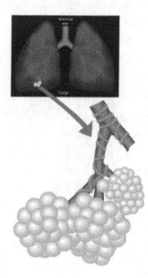

Standard textbooks must take the blame for misleading us and misrepresenting the anatomy of the lungs when they described the alveoli as of equal size and structured "like a bunch of grapes." The figure represents a misconception of anatomy and misapplication of physics.

Newtonian physics and the size of our alveoli

Newton concluded that the same force influenced the apple and the moon. He named that force gravitation (or gravity) after the Latin word *gravitas*, which means "heaviness" or "weight." Newton expressed this concept in a simple equation in which F is the force between two masses, G is the gravitational constant, m is mass and r is the distance between the centres of the masses.

$$F = G\frac{m_1 m_2}{r^2}$$

As we carry our lungs in an erect posture, these gravitational forces affect both blood flow in the lungs and the size of our alveoli. In the upright (vertical) lung, there are three functional zones into which the distribution of blood flow can be divided. **Zone 1** is the uppermost portion of the lung. In it, the air pressure in the alveoli is higher than the pulmonary arterial pressure so blood flow is obstructed, and as a result, there is little or no blood flow at rest. In **zone 2**, the pulmonary arterial pressure is greater than the pulmonary alveolar pressure so that there is low to moderate flow. In the bottom third of the upright lung, know as **zone 3**, pulmonary arterial pressure is greater than both alveolar and venous pressure, and as a result, there is high blood flow in this part of the lung. This would be perfect if airflow in the bottom of the lung were also high, so that the efficiency of exchange of oxygen and carbon dioxide between blood and air were maximized. This can happen only if the alveoli in the bottom third of the lung 'breathe' more or, at least, expand and contract more than in the top third of the lung. Gravity ensures this is precisely what happens.

Slinky and the lung

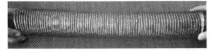

Imagine that gravity affects the size of alveoli in a similar manner to the way it affects the distances between the coils of a slinky. Place the slinky horizontally on a firm surface and expand it a little. Observe that the spaces representing the alveoli are all approximately the same size.

Slinky exhaling

Now hold the slinky vertically, like an erect lung, and observe the effect of gravity. The slinky represents how the alveoli appear at the end of breathing out, that is to say, at the point of maximal exhalation.

Observe how the alveoli at the top are much larger than at the bottom, gradually decreasing in volume as we descend to the bottom of the lung, where many of the alveoli are completely closed.

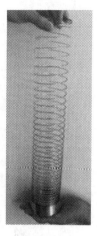

Slinky inhaling

Now imagine inhaling. This is achieved by contraction of the diaphragm, which by flattening out pulls the bottom of the lungs down.

In our slinky model, we will simulate a breath in by holding the upper hand steady and pulling the slinky down with our lower hand. What happens? The whole lung expands.

The 'alveoli' in the lower third of the lung expand and those that were nearly closed when breathing out open up, but the big ones at the top of the lung hardly change size.

In other words:

1. Alveoli in the upper third of the lung have a bigger volume than those at the bottom of the lung.

2. During breathing, the alveoli at the bottom of the lung change much more in size than do the big alveoli at the top of the lung.

3. Because of gravity, blood flow at the bottom of the lung is much higher than at the top, so that air going in and out (ventilation) matches beautifully with blood flow (perfusion).

4. At the top of the lung, where alveoli do not change their size during breathing, there is almost no blood flow, and therefore no "wasted" perfusion.

5. Hence, the matching of ventilation and blood flow in the normal, healthy lung ensures the maximum efficiency of transferring oxygen from the air we breathe to the blood.

Laplace's law and the size of our alveoli

If big alveoli are connected to small alveoli, though, why do they not equalize like a nice uniform bunch of grapes?

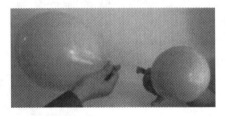

The answer to that question is partly to be found in Laplace's law, which states that the pressure inside an inflated elastic container with a curved surface is inversely proportional to the radius as long as the surface tension is relatively uniform throughout the surface. A common illustration of this phenomenon is the effort required to blow up a balloon: it is greatest when the diameter of the balloon is at its smallest. Thus, if we inflate a balloon until it is big and connect it to a balloon that is less inflated, what do you think happens? According to the theory underlying the "bunch of grapes" image, one would presume that the two balloons equalized in size, with air from the larger balloon flowing into the smaller balloon.

Wrong!

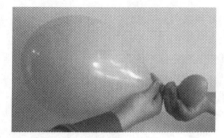

According to Laplace's law, because the radius of the small balloon is less than the radius of the big balloon, the tension in the wall of the small balloon is greater than that of the big balloon. Hence, the small balloon empties into the big balloon

This, however, raises a further problem: if the alveoli are of unequal size, according to Laplace's law all the small alveoli would empty into the larger alveoli and our lungs would collapse. They do not, of course.

Why not?

There are at least two reasons that the lungs remain stable and do **not**, under normal conditions, obey Laplace's law.

The first reason is because the small airways that connect the alveoli and the alveolar walls are coated with an amazing substance called surfactant, which alters the surface tension of the alveoli of different radii so that, so that the alveoli are no longer totally under the influence of Laplace's law.

The other main reasons why the small alveoli do not collapse are that the alveoli are not independent of one another and they do not have curved, much less spherical, walls. Each alveolus shares walls in common with adjacent alveoli. The patency of the alveoli, that is to say keeping alveoli inflated, is maintained by the tension through the connective tissue of the lung. Although regions or lobes of the lung may be partially collapsed, one alveolus cannot readily collapse into another because it is not held inflated simply by positive pressure like a balloon. Rather, the alveoli are held in place by a connective tissue framework. Last but not least, unlike grapes, there are pores in the walls of the alveoli, connecting the alveoli that share common walls.

Anthony Rebuck

A final word on surfactant

Although there are several factors that prevent Laplace's law from simply controlling the size and functioning of alveoli, surfactant is the most important factor. Without it, Laplace's law would cause the small alveoli to empty into the large ones. Small alveoli would close and the larger ones expand further. Because surfactant stabilizes the surface tension of the inner linings of the alveoli, it is fundamental to the stability and functioning of healthy lungs.

Pulmonary surfactant is a phospho-lipoprotein complex, produced by alveolar cells. The surfactant molecule has a hydrophilic region and a hydrophobic region. The main lipid component of surfactant is responsible for reducing surface tension and hence stabilizing the alveoli and regulating their size.

Surfactant in the lungs also has an immune function. The protein part of the surfactant molecule binds to sugars on the surface of bacterial pathogens, making them more easily ingested by phagocytic cells. If the surfactant is degraded or inactivated in any way, the lung is rendered more susceptible to inflammation and infection.

A lack of surfactant, as one can imagine, is potentially fatal. Infant respiratory distress syndrome (IRDS), for example, can occur in babies born before 28 weeks of gestation, which is before surfactant is present in the lungs. In these premature babies, the alveoli do not expand until they start to produce surfactant. Corticosteroids increase surfactant production in premature babies. This is the reason why corticosteroids are given to expectant mothers who are at risk of early delivery and why premature babies are often given one or more doses of artificial surfactant to help their lungs stay open.

Last but not least, a further harmful effect of smoking has been identified:

There is now strong evidence that surfactant levels are reduced in smokers and in patients with COPD.

Lung surfactant forms a single molecular layer film that reduces the effort required to breathe by more than 90% (compared to the energy required without the layer). In other words, without functional lung surfactant, normal breathing is impossible. The surfactant layer is also one of the first lines of defence against lung injury and disease. What happens when this layer is exposed to tobacco smoke? Researchers in the University of California (Sazadzinski, 1997) have constructed a lung model with a surfactant layer. When they exposed this layer to the oxidants in tobacco smoke, they observed a disruption of the lipid structure in their surfactant model.

While the precise effects of smoking on surfactant structure and function are unknown, these observations raise the possibility that some of the harmful effects of tobacco might be through a disruption of surfactant—the extraordinary phospholipid that ensures efficient functioning of our alveoli.

CHAPTER 5

Is COPD Fatal?

According to the American College of Chest Physicians, COPD is responsible for more than 2.5 million deaths worldwide each year. In a recent Danish study reported at the European Respiratory Society's annual meeting, the average survival time in patients with COPD was 10.4 years. Age and the "pack-year" smoking history were significant predictors of mortality. The third strongly significant predictive factor was the degree of emphysema as measured by CT scan.

Patients with COPD can be divided broadly into two clinically recognizable groups: those with predominant emphysema and a second group whose disease has a major chronic bronchitis component. Patients in the first group are characteristically thin with wasted muscles and short of breath; they are referred to as "pink puffers." Patients in the second group—"the blue bloaters"—are typically overweight rather than underweight, have a productive cough and frequently have a blue tinge of cyanosis in their lips. The causes of death in the two groups are usually quite different.

Anthony Rebuck

Pink Puffers

In pink puffers, the underlying pathology is primarily emphysema. These are patients in whom the ravages of smoke and noxious particles have caused elastic tissue in the lungs to break down, which in turn causes a loss of alveolar wall integrity. The destruction of alveoli is accompanied by—and may indeed be preceded by—the narrowing and disappearance of tiny terminal bronchioles that supply the alveoli. This pathological picture characterizes centrilobular emphysema. It is usually apparent in smokers in the sixth or seventh decade of life, but it can occur much earlier in people with alpha-1 antitrypsin deficiency, where the pathology is more characteristically pan-lobular emphysema.

In emphysema, as the terminal bronchioles and alveoli are destroyed, the blood vessels are destroyed, too. This reduces the area for gas exchange, i.e., the process of getting oxygen in and carbon dioxide out. The alveoli disappear, as do the capillaries that supply them. Because ventilation and perfusion are destroyed at the same time, however, the ratio between them is relatively well preserved, and the patient can compensate by breathing hard (puffing) and hyperventilating the remaining alveoli. Through this increased work of breathing, the patient manages to maintain relatively normal levels of oxygen and carbon dioxide in his or her blood (which therefore appears pink). The loss of blood vessels in the lungs, however, increases the resistance to flow in the remaining vessels, throwing a load on the right ventricle of the heart, which now has to work harder to deliver sufficient cardiac output to the lungs. Pink puffers thus work hard for every breath; they puff away using every muscle available to keep their chests pumping. Even the neck muscles attached to their upper ribs are used. The extra work they must do just to draw a breath usually results in weight loss.

The increased work that the heart must do to pump blood through the lungs frequently leads to strain of the heart muscle and eventually failure of the right side of the heart, a condition known as *cor pulmonale,* or pulmonary heart disease. The walls of the right ventricle at first thicken to fight the increased resistance in the blood vessels in the lungs, and then, as the ventricle starts to fail, it dilates. Gradually, blood starts to back up in the veins, the liver becomes congested, and the ankles and abdomen become swollen due to fluid accumulation (ascites). Death is most commonly due to cardiac failure, usually following an acute respiratory infection.

Blue Bloaters

In blue bloaters, the underlying pathology is primarily chronic bronchitis. In chronic bronchitis, smoke and noxious particles target the airways instead of the alveoli. The smoke induces excessive mucous production and enlarges the mucous-producing glands in the bronchi. The bronchi become inflamed, and inflammatory cells such as neutrophils pack the walls of the airways. As the walls of the bronchi swell and thicken with inflammatory fluid, cells and debris, the lumen of the tubes narrows. It is this obstruction to airflow that characterizes COPD. In contrast to emphysema, when the airways become narrowed so that ventilation through them is impaired, the blood vessels escape damage. The result is a complete mismatch between ventilation and perfusion. The blood flow is "wasted" as it goes through the lungs and bypasses areas where gas exchange might have taken place. Gradually the carbon dioxide in the body accumulates and levels of CO_2 increase in the blood. Breathing slows down. Because of the effect of CO_2 on red blood cells, (in technical terms, the oxyhemoglobin dissociation curve is shifted to the right) the cells become less efficient at carrying what little oxygen the lungs are supplying. That is to say, the cells become desaturated. Desaturated haemoglobin loses its characteristic red colour and becomes blue, rather like venous blood—hence, the blue cyanotic colour of patients with chronic bronchitis. As airways narrow, gas (air) gets trapped in the lungs, the trapped gas increases the volume of the lungs, and this increased volume, together with the fluid retention caused by the abnormal blood gases, gives the patient a bloated appearance.

Chronic bronchitis does not damage the lungs as much as emphysema does, but the pathology in the major airways is severe. The bronchi become blocked by mucous plugs and narrowed by inflammation in their walls. Patients are subject to recurrent acute exacerbations of respiratory infections, sometimes many times a year, and frequently require hospitalization. After an acute exacerbation, it is exceedingly rare for a patient to recover to the same level of lung function as before the episode. More than 10% die during acute relapses, and over half of those who do recover return to the hospital within six months. Death during hospital admissions is more commonly due to respiratory failure than to heart failure, although the chronic levels of low oxygen impair cardiac function in many patients. Unfortunately, and hardly surprisingly, anxiety and depression frequently occur when patients find that they can no longer walk or perform even the most basic activities of daily living.

The smoking that causes COPD is also associated with a high risk of pneumonia, lung cancer, stroke and heart attack. Most patients with COPD experience sleep disorders, such as obstructive sleep apnoea, with profound, life-threatening falls in blood oxygen.

In summary, COPD is fatal and is rapidly becoming the third leading cause of death in the world. There is, of course, an overlap between chronic bronchitis and emphysema, and the causes of death therefore overlap between cardiac and respiratory failure.

CHAPTER 6

How Common is COPD in Asia?

COPD in Asia is a gathering storm. All previous efforts to estimate the numbers have failed to take into account the combined impacts of smoking, pollution and haze in trying to calculate how many people in Asia might have COPD and, accordingly, have severely underestimated the extent of the disease. A likely estimate is well in excess of 100 million. In Asia, COPD is rarely diagnosed in its early stages. Chronic cough, for example, is frequently deemed an innocent accompaniment of smoking or simply a manifestation of ageing. Although descriptions in the Asian medical literature of "voluminous lungs," "distended air sacks" and cough with mucous have existed for centuries and the condition was described as disabling as long ago as 1814, Asia has lagged behind in recognizing the symptoms as a real disease; the term COPD was introduced in some Asian countries only as recently as 1995. As Professor Buist would say, "COPD doesn't get much sympathy (or for that matter a lot of research funding), largely because as a smoker's problem, it is considered to be self-inflicted."

The problem in extrapolating COPD numbers in Asia from global statistics is that most of the information on COPD prevalence, morbidity and mortality comes from developed, high-income countries. Yet, according to the World Health Organization (WHO)—and here is the irony—90% of COPD deaths occur in low and middle-income countries.

The first step in trying to estimate COPD numbers is to agree on a definition, and unfortunately, there are many from which to choose. The Global Initiative for Chronic Lung Disease (GOLD) defines COPD as "a disease state characterized by airflow limitation that is not fully reversible. The airflow limitation is usually progressive and is associated with an abnormal inflammatory response of the lungs to noxious particles or gases." The key to this definition is that airflow limitation has to be demonstrated—by lung function testing—in order to make the diagnosis correctly. The GOLD definition of airflow limitation is an FEV_1/FVC ratio of less than 70%, where FEV_1 is the forced expired volume in the first second of an exhalation. The FVC is the forced vital capacity which is blowing out as hard as one can, until no more air comes out,—the simplest and most widely accepted of all lung function tests.

The National Health Interview Surveys of prevalence of COPD in the United States in the 1990s perfectly illustrate how the numbers come out when the GOLD definition is not used. Data collection was at that time achieved just by asking people whether they had had any respiratory diseases in the last twelve months, and, if so, what kind. Simply adding together the numbers for chronic bronchitis and emphysema arrived at the COPD prevalence calculation in 1996 of 11.9 million.

The National Health and Nutrition Examination Survey was much more thorough. Participants completed questionnaires and had physical examinations and lung-function testing. This time the estimated national prevalence estimation was a more realistic 23.6 million or 13.9% of the adult population. One astonishing statistic from this study was that 63% of the study population with clear GOLD-standard evidence of COPD had never previously had a diagnosis of lung disease. The conclusion appears obvious: a large proportion of adults with COPD are completely unrecognized as having a pulmonary medical condition. (Some of these patients might have had asthma rather than COPD or combined asthma and COPD, but this possibility could not be evaluated, as reversibility of their airways obstruction with bronchodilators was not measured.)

Irrespective of statistical design details, methods of evaluation and strict criteria for diagnosis, all of the many studies in the literature on epidemiology lead to the same conclusion: the prevalence of COPD is increasing. The main reason for underestimating the worldwide prevalence is the delay in performing pulmonary function tests and thereby establishing a diagnosis after the onset of cough and shortness of breath. There are other problems, of course, such as the variability in definitions of COPD and the lack of age-adjusted estimates. Age adjustment is important because the prevalence of COPD in people under the age of 45 is low while in people over the age of 65 it is several times higher. Yet another impediment is that older studies were conducted mainly on men, but we now know that the gender distribution of COPD is changing. Deaths from COPD in women now exceed those in men.

Just how rapidly predictions for the burden and impact of COPD are changing can be appreciated from WHO's 1996 estimates. In 1996, WHO estimated that COPD would rise from the seventh-leading cause of death and disability worldwide to fifth position by 2020. COPD has achieved this awful ranking seven years ahead of schedule. Currently, the revised prediction is for COPD to achieve third place among the causes of death by 2020.

In a paper in the *Lancet* in 2003, Professor Calverley and Dr. Walker, both from Liverpool, predicted correctly the rise in COPD that was about to occur. In their paper, however, they made no distinction between Asian countries, on the one hand, and European and North American countries, on the other hand. Increasingly, physicians in Canada are beginning to report that much of the increase in COPD prevalence will occur in Asia. Yet, despite high rates of cigarette smoking and widespread use of biomass fuels, there are few objective data on the prevalence of COPD in the region.

A revised estimate of the number of patients with COPD in Asia

How can we justify predicting a prevalence of COPD in Asia of 100 million, a number that is approximately double in the current estimate in the medical literature?

Our basic assumptions are widely accepted by specialists in the field:

1. COPD is a chronic, progressive disorder caused by cigarette smoking, exposure to biomass smoke and other forms of pollution.
2. Airway narrowing and obstruction decrease lung function in COPD patients.
3. COPD results in death or disability.
4. Because of lack of awareness and inadequate access to lung-function testing, the disease is largely hidden, and less than half the patients who have COPD are diagnosed with it.

The current estimate of the number of patients with moderate to severe COPD in the Asia-Pacific countries is 56.6 million. A Regional COPD Working Group derived this estimate from a study in 2003 with representatives from Singapore, Australia, Thailand, the Philippines, China, Indonesia and South Korea. Twelve Asian countries were studied using a validated, computerized tool that employed epidemiological relationships and risk-factor prevalence to project COPD numbers in given populations aged 30 years and older. According to the Working Group, in Singapore and Hong Kong COPD prevalence rates were 3.5%. In Vietnam, the Group reported a prevalence rate of 6.7% and overall—and here is the big problem—a prevalence rate of 6.3% for the region as a whole. Although this figure is much higher than the WHO estimate of 3.8%, it is almost certainly wrong.

The authors of the study point out that in the WHO Burden of Disease study in 1979, estimates were divided into three categories: established market economies, former socialist economies of Europe and a third category called demographically developed regions, which included China, India and "other Asian Islands." As Professor Tan of Singapore pointed out, Asia-Pacific received insufficient focus, to say the least. Asia is distinct in many ways. It is economically, socially and geographically diverse, with some countries boasting established market economies such as Japan, Singapore and Australia, and others having developing markets, such as many of the nations in Southeast and East Asia. Furthermore, it is a region that is experiencing rapidly changing demographics, lifestyle and disease patterns.

The estimated overall prevalence of 6.3% for COPD in the twelve countries surveyed is different from the WHO extrapolated data, but a closer examination of the estimate is surely justified, especially since the 2003 study did not include India. Furthermore, if the global prevalence of physiologically defined COPD in adults aged 40 years or more is 9-10%, as noted earlier, how on earth could the prevalence in polluted, cigarette-smoking Asia be so much less? At the very least, just as a simple statistical calculation, the number must be closer to 89 million. The question now arises as to whether the global estimate of 10% is applicable to Asia, which, to say nothing of haze, is the most polluted and highest cigarette-consuming region of the world.

Take, for example, India and Pakistan. These countries were not included among the 12 countries in the Asia prevalence study. (The countries were Australia, China, Hong Kong, Indonesia, Japan, South Korea, Malaysia, Philippines, Singapore,

Taiwan, Thailand and Vietnam.) India and Pakistan are now infamous for containing, according to *science.time.com,* five of the most polluted cities in the world (Ludhiana, Kanpor and Mumbai in India, and Quetta and Peshawar in Pakistan). Dr. S.K. Jindal of the WHO Collaborating Centre for Research in Chandigarh calls COPD in India an unrecognized epidemic. In some studies in India, astonishing prevalence rates as high as 22% in men and 19% in women have been recorded based on questionnaire interviews. Other studies conducted by the Indian Medical Research Council reported the much lower figure of five per cent in Delhi and Bangalore. However, in some rural areas such as Maharashtra, where there is a higher level of indoor air pollution from combustion of solid fuels for cooking as well as from exposure to passive smoking in the home, COPD is the leading cause of death. Physicians in India, reports Dr Jindal, are generally dismissive of the progressive and disabling nature of COPD and frequently ignore it as simple bronchitis and, hence, as inconsequential and insignificant. Management of COPD in India rarely follows the GOLD guidelines, and rehabilitation is non-existent. Rarely do patients receive any specific COPD medications, and if treated, they are likely to be given nothing more than cough suppressants, cough expectorants and antibiotics.

Teams from Imperial College, London and JSS University in Mysore have conducted a systematic review of 351 publications reporting the prevalence of COPD/chronic bronchitis in India. Their conclusion is that "the current prevalence of COPD in India is unclear." Nevertheless, they found one report in which the prevalence of airways obstruction was 58.5%, although symptoms were not recorded so the data may have included patients with asthma. Some studies showed well-documented chronic bronchitis rates of 20.9% in rural communities, and others showed rates as low as 9.1% in some urban areas. Irrespective of any shortcomings in the available data, the following seems inescapable: first, the presence of COPD/

chronic bronchitis in India is great; second, COPD will increase; and third, the Asian estimate of 6.3% prevalence significant underestimates the problem.

Just suppose, for the sake of argument, that the prevalence rate of COPD in Asia really is 6.3%. Then India, with 17.5% of the world's population and 1.21 billion residents, would have 76.2 million people with COPD.

In that case, how can we accept without challenging a prediction of 56.6 million? This makes no sense, especially since we have not yet taken China into account.

One does not have to be a smoker in China to develop COPD. The Guangzhou Medical University recently conducted an epidemiological survey of 20,245 subjects aged 40 years or older, using questionnaires and lung-function testing. The survey found an overall prevalence of COPD among non-smokers of 5.2%. Being male, of advanced age, lower body mass index and lower educational level, being exposed to second-hand tobacco smoke, coal or other biomass smoke, having poor ventilation in the kitchen and a childhood cough—all these factors were independently associated with a higher risk of COPD among non-smokers.

Then there are the smokers. At least two thirds of men in China smoke, but only 4% of women do.

One third of all the cigarettes in the world are smoked in China, and the number of smokers in China is estimated at approximately 300 million. China is now the largest producer of tobacco and, what is more, is in partnership with their government.

The current estimate for prevalent cases of COPD in China is 42 million. This is predicted to increase to nearly 56 million by the year 2020. Why? Because in China COPD is a disease of the aged; of the 42 million people diagnosed with COPD at the present time, most cases are above the age of 60. As for India, though, this figure of 42 million is undoubtedly low.

Let us turn to other Asian countries. Professor Ali Zubairi of Aga Khan University in Karachi has written that in Pakistan, COPD is under-diagnosed and under-treated. At least ten per cent of the adult population over the age of 40, he estimates, has the disease.

Indonesia, with over 238 million people, is the world's fourth most populous country, and in it, 63% of men are smokers. Indonesia is the fifth largest tobacco market in the world, and every year, approximately 160 billion cigarettes are sold. Most of the smokers also use kretek cigarettes, which are cigarettes that combine tobacco, cloves, cocoa and dry cornhusk. The concentration of tar and nicotine in these cigarettes is almost four times higher than in regular cigarettes. In Indonesia, the tobacco industry is thriving. More than 30% of children have their first cigarette before the age of ten, and one infamous child in Sumatra made global headlines for having a 40-a-day cigarette habit at the age of two! (His father had initiated him into the habit at the age of 18 months.) Needless to say, the tobacco industry targets young people; cigarette advertising and promotion was recently estimated to be valued at US$250 million. There is no ban on smoking in government or private offices, restaurants or bars. How could it possibly be correct that the rate of moderate to severe cases of COPD in Indonesia, originators of the notorious haze, is only 5.6%, or 4.8 million?

Indonesia's neighbour Malaysia takes smoking far more seriously. Warning messages have been appearing on cigarette packages since 1976. Smoking has been banned in public places since 1980 and tobacco advertising is completely banned. The quoted prevalence of 4.7% for COPD is therefore much easier to accept than the rate attributed to Indonesia.

In the Philippines, 18.7% of women smoke and 30% of all girls between 15-23 years smoke regularly. Pollution is so bad in Manila that pulmonary doctors advise all visitors to live by the sea to avoid vehicular exhaust, smoke from wood stoves and daily burning of household trash. A recent study was conducted by researchers of the Lung Centre of the Philippines on people living in the Nueva Ecija province. They used the strict criteria of the Burden of Obstructive Lung Disease (BOLD) protocol and study design, which includes lung-function testing. The prevalence of COPD was 20.8%. In men, the prevalence was as high as 26.5% and was strongly related to a history of smoking and tuberculosis, the use of firewood for cooking, and working on a farm.

The age-adjusted death rate is 29.10 per 100,000 of population ranks Philippines #76 in the world.

In Australia, COPD is known as a hidden disease. The current estimate is that almost 13% of Australians over the age of 40, or one in seven, have COPD. Approximately half of these people who have lost 50% of their lung function do not know that they have COPD. Therefore, they do not seek (or receive) appropriate medical treatment to slow down disease progression. They consider their symptoms, such as breathlessness, a natural sign of ageing.

In summary, a COPD prevalence of 56.6 million people in the Asia-Pacific region is shockingly low. Millions more people are living with a preventable, disabling, incurable disease.

Indeed, the number is frankly laughable. It is a mystery as to why it has been so widely accepted. Just combining the numbers for China and India alone when applying the worldwide prevalence rate of 6.3% yields a figure of 119,300,000 people with COPD.

COPD thus continues to be under-diagnosed, under-treated and underestimated. Sam Lim of the Duke NUS Graduate School of Medicine in Singapore calls COPD in Asia an epidemic time bomb that may explode if urgent actions are not taken to curb the trend. The poorer countries of the Asia-Pacific region simply cannot afford the economic burden of hospitalizations and lost productivity. Professor Price of Adelaide agrees and says that Asia is experiencing "a massive increase in COPD due to smoking and longer life spans."

CHAPTER 7

Management of COPD: Smoking Cessation, Oxygen, Surgery and Rehabilitation

It is a sobering thought that after a professional life-time working in research and development of drugs for patients with COPD, this author must admit that not a single drug or combination of drugs has a proven influence on mortality. Indeed, age-adjusted death rates continue to increase year-by-year and have almost doubled since 1979. Furthermore, COPD mortality rates in Asian countries are markedly higher than in Western Europe and the USA, largely as a result of smoking, pollution, haze and infectious diseases. The death rates in Asia might be even higher than suspected, as they are under-reported due to under-diagnosis of the disease.

Studies of safe, efficacious drugs such as long-acting bronchodilators, inhaled corticosteroids, combination inhalers, oral steroids, phosphodiesterase inhibitors and antibiotics show no difference in survival rates between treatment and placebo. This is not to say that the drugs do not bring tremendous relief of symptoms, improved recovery rates from acute exacerbations, reduced numbers of hospital admissions and improved quality of life. They do, and they do it well, but none results in patients living longer (although the anticholinergic drug tiotropium comes tantalizingly close, as does a combination of fluticasone and salmeterol—close, but the measured improvements are not quite statistically significant enough).

The goals of management of COPD are to slow disease progression, relieve symptoms, improve exercise tolerance, prevent and treat acute exacerbations and, last but not least, reduce mortality. Only two actions consistently and significantly improve life expectancy in patients with COPD: smoking cessation and long-term oxygen therapy.

Smoking cessation

Professor Charles Fletcher spent his life investigating and educating his medical colleagues on lung disease. Thirty-five years ago, he and his co-author R. Peto reported in the British Medical Journal, the results of their measurements of the forced expiratory volume in one second (FEV_1), the simplest of all lung-function tests, every six months over an eight-year period in a cohort of 792 men. Their iconic graph showed the decline in FEV_1 over time in COPD patients compared with healthy subjects. The lessons learned from this landmark study concerned individual susceptibility to smoking-related lung function damage and the unavoidable progressive decline once airflow obstruction begins. The seminal observation was the reduction in the rate of FEV_1 decline after smoking cessation.

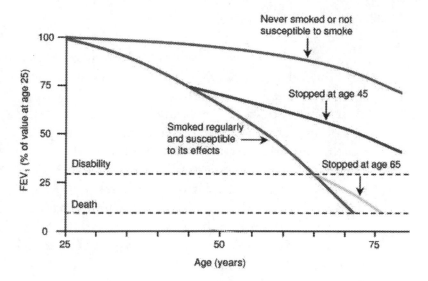

Now, decades later, researchers are mildly critical of these somewhat simplistic curves, which had been extrapolated backwards and forwards to compensate for the relatively short follow-up period and the fact that the study subjects were all between 30 and 59 years old. The risk in over-interpreting the Fletcher and Peto graph is that it gives an impression that COPD progresses slowly early on in its course, then speeds up only when a certain degree of airway narrowing has occurred. Accordingly, some physicians may interpret the shape of the curve as suggesting that intensive treatment is only worthwhile when COPD is severe and well advanced. Recent studies are now showing that the late accelerated decline is not an accurate interpretation of the natural history. Tantucci and Modina from the University of Brescia in Italy (2012) have collected evidence from a number of studies that now indicate that the loss of lung function is in fact more accelerated in the early stages of COPD than in the late stages. Patients in early stages of COPD therefore have more to lose than those in the late stages and should therefore have more to benefit from early intervention.

The message is loud and clear:

1. Screen for COPD in susceptible **young people**, i.e., smokers and those exposed to excessive pollution and industrial fumes.
2. Obtain lung-function data early in the course of the disease and repeat at regular intervals to follow progress.
3. Start therapeutic intervention as early as possible.
4. Do everything possible to discourage smoking and encourage quitting, the **earlier the better**! Quitting at the age of 30 reduces the chance of dying prematurely from smoking-related diseases by more than 90%. Quitting at 50 halves the risk. Even if people quit at 60 or older, according to Doll, Boreham and Sutherland's article in the *British Medical Journal* in 2004, they will live longer than those who continues to smoke.

Quitting smoking: Is it really worth all the mental suffering and weight gain?

What factors contribute to a person's learning to smoke, continuing to smoke and then having difficulty quitting? There appears to be a connection between genetics and nicotine addiction, and researchers have been focusing on various genetic regions believed to be involved in one's vulnerability to addiction. Some have studied genes that control certain neurotransmitters in the brain, while others have looked at genes related to addictive traits like risk-taking and impulsiveness. The studies indicate that variations in specific genes substantially increase the risk of addiction, affect susceptibility to adverse health effects and even affect whether smoking cessation medications will help.

A number of studies have shown that women have more difficulty quitting and are less likely to quit than men. Perhaps they are genetically programmed to experience the symptoms and physiology of withdrawal differently, or perhaps medications designed to help quitting may not work in women. In addition, some women are very concerned about gaining weight, and indeed, weight gain is common after quitting smoking, although most of the time, the weight gain is not excessive. Combining quitting with changes in diet and increased exercise mitigates the quitting-induced weight gain in most cases. Even if weight gain does result, the benefits from smoking cessation manifestly outweigh the harms from weight gain.

First, smoking cessation is the single most effective way to reduce the risk of developing COPD. It is the only intervention proven to slow the accelerated decline in lung function related to chronic obstructive pulmonary disease. Smoking cessation also reduces mortality rates even in those with established symptoms of COPD. In a 14-year follow up of the Lung Health Study of 6000 smokers with symptomatic airway obstruction (Anthonisen, 1994; Decramer, 2005), those who underwent an intensive 10-week smoking cessation intervention program reduced all-cause mortality compared with controls who did not participate in the program. Even more important was the finding that there was a reduction in respiratory deaths that was both clinically and statistically significant.

There are also other benefits from smoking cessation. What are they and how quickly do they appear? Answer: the benefits are immediate. The elevations of heart rate and blood pressure associated with smoking begin to return to normal immediately. Within minutes, the level of carbon monoxide in the blood starts to decline. The half-life of carbon monoxide in the body when we breathe air is five hours, so it takes 12 hours for carbon monoxide to leave the body completely after a cigarette is smoked, provided that one does not smoke another cigarette and is not exposed to second-hand smoke during the 12 hours.

Within two weeks to three months after quitting, the risk of heart attack begins to decrease and lung function starts to improve, especially in the small airways, many of which have been completely closed by inflammation and swelling in their walls. Over the next six months, almost all ex-smokers notice a reduction or even complete disappearance of their cough and much less shortness of breath. By the end of the first year, the risk of coronary heart disease will have fallen to that of a lifetime non-smoker's. Over the next very few years, the risks of having a stroke and of getting cancer of the mouth, throat, lung, bladder, kidney or pancreas will also be that of a lifetime non-smoker.

As for the so-called perils of weight gain, a study funded by the U.S. National Institutes of Health (NIH) has recently reported that former smokers had about half as much risk of developing cardiovascular disease as current smokers. Furthermore, the risk level did not change when post-cessation weight gain was taken into account. In other words, the improvement in cardiovascular health that results from quitting smoking outweighs the limited risks to cardiovascular health from the modest amount of weight gained after quitting; the benefits of quitting smoking more than balance the risk of modest weight gain.

Oxygen.

As noted earlier, while there is no cure for COPD, the disease is preventable and treatable, and only two things have been shown to reduce mortality from COPD: (1) smoking cessation, which can never happen too late and which provides the greatest benefits early in the disease and (2) oxygen, usually reserved for the late, advanced stages. Let us now turn to oxygen.

Supplemental oxygen is given to COPD patients when their blood oxygen is low at rest, when their oxygen levels fall precipitously during exertion, or when their arterial oxygen saturation levels plummet during the night.

What is oxygen, and why does administering supplemental oxygen help patients with COPD live longer?

Students in biology class learn that living green plants use sunlight to make glucose from carbon dioxide and water. During this process, known as photosynthesis, oxygen is liberated. In nature there is no source of oxygen other than green algae in the ocean and plants on land. The air we breathe contains 20.8% oxygen, the rest is mainly nitrogen. Nitrogen is a building block of amino acids and nucleic acids in our bodies, and it is essential to life on earth, but the nitrogen we breathe from the atmosphere cannot be used by us, or by plants or by animals, as it is completely inert. We have to obtain our nitrogen from bacteria and the nitrates and nitrites in what we eat. Oxygen, on the other hand, which is necessary to sustain almost all terrestrial life, comes to us from only one source and in only one form that we can use, the air we breathe.

Oxygen passes from air into the capillaries that line the alveoli in the lungs by a passive process, simply because the pressure of oxygen in air is greater than the pressure of oxygen in the lungs. Let us assume that we are at sea level and the barometric pressure today is 760 mm Hg. We know that the air surrounding us is mainly nitrogen but 20.8% of it is oxygen. 20.8% of 760 is 158. That means the pressure of oxygen in air is 158 mm Hg. The pressure of oxygen in the alveoli depends partly on the pressure of oxygen in the venous blood arriving in the lungs from the body tissues and partly on water vapour. On average, the pressure of oxygen in the alveoli is 110 mm Hg. There is therefore a gradient of pressure from 158 to 110, so that as long as we continue to breathe, oxygen passes passively into the blood lining the alveoli.

Now the most interesting point of all is that our bodies have absolutely no ability to store oxygen, which means that to stay alive and function, our tissues depend on a continuous supply. As a result, oxygen transport in the blood needs to be very energy-efficient so that the oxygen supply can meet demand, both at rest and during exercise. Blood must release oxygen rapidly upon arrival in the tissues, and it is critical that there be minimal waste or loss during transmission. The fact of the matter is that oxygen is not very soluble in blood. In the entire 5 litres of blood that the average human body possesses, only 15 ml of oxygen are dissolved, yet we consume around 250 ml every minute, even sitting quietly at rest. Clearly, if survival depended on the amount of oxygen dissolved in blood, we would not survive! We need some way to increase the oxygen levels in our blood, and that is where haemoglobin comes in. Haemoglobin increases oxygen transport almost a hundred-fold so that 98% of oxygen is attached to haemoglobin and a mere 2% dissolved in plasma. Many factors such as temperature, carbon dioxide and acidity can affect how the haemoglobin functions. One that is very relevant for our purposes, and worth mentioning here, is that carbon monoxide binds to haemoglobin **230 times** more efficiently than oxygen. Carbon monoxide, a significant component of cigarette smoke, motor vehicle pollution and home heaters, pushes oxygen off haemoglobin. It is one of the major poisons we breathe.

In COPD blood oxygen levels are reduced (this is called hypoxemia) because the obstruction of the bronchi (breathing tubes) in the lungs causes a mismatch between breathing and blood flow in the lungs. Technically, and as noted earlier, this is known as a ventilation/perfusion inequality. In some areas of the smoke-ravaged lungs of people with COPD, blood flows to the alveoli to pick up a fresh load of oxygen, but the airway is blocked so that the blood flow is wasted. This is called a physiological shunt—the blood from those areas of the lung leave with the same amount of oxygen as when it arrived. In other areas, air comes to the alveoli, but destructive lung diseases such as emphysema have destroyed blood vessel walls. The result is wasted ventilation, often referred to as a physiological dead space. Think of it as waiting for a train that, when it finally arrives, does not stop at your platform. Although ventilation/perfusion mismatch is the main cause of hypoxemia in COPD, other factors can contribute. Obesity, for example, stiffens the chest wall and squashes small airways, and it is associated with sleep-related breathing disorders (sleep apnoea), which cause patients to reduce their breathing at night during periods and even to stop breathing altogether for a minute or so. A further factor in developing hypoxemia is the blunted response to the usual stimuli to increase our breathing, such as exercise, low oxygen in the air and raised carbon dioxide levels. Normal subjects have a brisk response to these chemical stimuli; patients with COPD lose this sensitivity.

The consequences of being hypoxemic are that the blood pressure in the lungs increases. Increased blood pressure in the lungs is a life-threatening condition known as pulmonary hypertension. The increased resistance to blood flow in the lungs throws a strain on the right side of the heart, which has to handle an increased workload, for which it is poorly designed. The strain under which the right ventricle must now labour is a contributor to the high incidence of heart failure as a cause of death in COPD patients.

Hypoxemia causes several other problems. Hypoxemic patients develop a condition known as polycythaemia, in which red blood cell numbers increase to compensate for the low levels of oxygen in the blood. While increased red cell counts are a putative advantage in competitive sports (such as the Tour de France), the result in patients with COPD, on balance, is negative. The thickened, sluggish blood with its extra red cells worsens the pulmonary hypertension because the blood flows poorly through the lungs. The blood flow to the brain decreases, and the increased red cells cause gout and easy clotting, the forerunners of venous thrombosis and pulmonary embolism.

Aside from smoking cessation, the most important intervention that prolongs the survival of patients with serious COPD is long-term oxygen therapy (LTOT). The statistics show clearly that in patients with severe resting arterial hypoxemia, LTOT reduces mortality. One might speculate that when patients come under the care of efficient providers who are monitoring the oxygen therapy, they may also be more likely to receive the timely benefits of pneumococcal and influenza vaccines, hospitalizations and intensive management of acute exacerbations and non-invasive positive-pressure ventilation. This multi-factorial care undoubtedly has a positive benefit in patients on LTOT, but the effect of oxygen itself is the major factor. Why?

Aside from the physiological reasons, oxygen therapy in patients with hypoxemia makes intuitive sense. Supplemental oxygen enhances blood oxygenation by increasing the percentage of oxygen in the inhaled air, thereby compensating for the ventilation/perfusion mismatch. Oxygen also regulates pulmonary blood flow; nothing reduces pulmonary vascular resistance as well as oxygen does. It acts like a potent drug, dilating the pulmonary vessels and (possibly by modulating gene expression) assisting in remodelling and repair in the lungs. The reasons for prescribing LTOT are based, according to published research, on improving mortality. Even before the mortality benefits were proven, it was well established that LTOT also could improve depression, cognitive function, quality of life and exercise tolerance, all of which are highly motivating for patients and important factors in acceptance and compliance.

Is LTOT, then, for everyone with COPD? No, it has not been established that patients with mild COPD derive benefits from LTOT, although it must be said that there is also no evidence of any harmful or adverse effects. In infants it is well recognised that high levels of oxygen and fluctuations in oxygen levels can cause retinopathy (eye damage). Perhaps increased levels of inhaled oxygen can produce increases in oxidative stress and hence stimulation of pathways that contribute to lung inflammation, but at present these are hypothetical issues that should be carefully evaluated in on-going research. The other negative considerations are cost, inconvenience and self-consciousness in social settings.

The costs relating to reimbursement of LTOT are measured in the billions of dollars. Approximately one third of all direct medical costs for COPD are due to the cost of LTOT, and 80% of this cost is borne by various medical care services such as Medicaid in the U.S. The cost is increasing at around 13% per year. Of course, the reimbursement for prescriptions is tightly regulated, and a close watch is being kept on the cost-effectiveness compared with other commonly used therapies for COPD. The current thinking is that LTOT for patients with severe COPD is indeed cost-effective, while nocturnal therapy alone is probably not. As Dr. Thomas L. Petty stated in the National Lung Health Education Program, LTOT is a bargain when compared with other technologies and surgeries used to extend life or improve the quality of life, but strict guidelines should be followed in prescribing long-term oxygen therapy for patients, and these should be restricted to those with advanced COPD.

1. The patient's condition should be stable on optimal medical therapy.
2. Arterial blood oxygen levels should be measured at least twice while the patient is breathing room air.
3. The arterial oxygen pressure should be less than 55 mm Hg.

As to how much oxygen is enough, there are also guidelines.

1. There should be continuous flow by double or single nasal cannula.
2. Use an oxygen delivery system that can be adjusted according to the level of oxygen saturation in the patient's blood.
3. Turn the oxygen delivery to the lowest level that raises the oxygen saturation to between 88% and 94%.
4. Increase the flow of oxygen during exercise and sleep.

Not so many years ago, after LTOT was prescribed, a patient would receive a visit from an industrial gas delivery supplier with several enormous gas cylinders. They would be placed in the bedroom and living areas as they would be much too cumbersome to be moved from place to place by the patient. Each tank would have a big metal regulator screwed into the top, as well as a humidifier since the gas was very dry and irritating to the nose. There were no portable systems. Then a device was developed that would generate oxygen in the home and never need to be refilled. These devices were called oxygen concentrators. The supply of oxygen was unlimited, provided of course there was no interruption of the electricity supply to power the concentrator. As a back-up, portable oxygen was made available in an emergency or if the patient needed to visit his health care provider or hospital clinic.

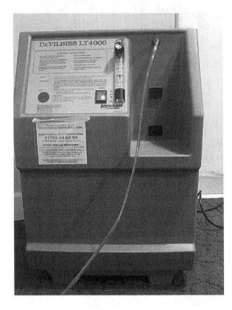

HOME OXYGEN CONCENTRATOR

Most portable oxygen concentrators today are the size of a binocular case and weigh less than a couple of 1kg (2 lb.) bags of sugar. The reason for this is because the on-demand system allows the concentrator to be built with smaller components. Since patients only inhale oxygen when they breathe in, when they breathe out, oxygen is wasted. By having the machine work with the patient's breathing cycle, only providing oxygen when necessary, the system keeps wasted oxygen to a minimum.

Over the years, cylinders have become lighter and more mobile, and the concentrators have become so small and light that patients can carry them with nothing more than a shoulder strap. The concentrators, by filling cylinders in the home, markedly reduce delivery costs. Air contains approximately 21% oxygen combined with nitrogen and a mixture of other gases. An air compressor inside the concentrator forces air through a system of chemical filters known as molecular sieves. The filter is made up of silicate granules, which remove nitrogen from the air, thereby concentrating the oxygen. Part of the oxygen produced is delivered to the patient, and part is fed back into the sieves to clear them of the accumulated nitrogen, preparing them for the next cycle. Through this process, the system is capable of producing medical grade oxygen of up to 96% consistently. The latest models can be powered from a wall socket in one's home, by 12v DC (as in a car or boat), and by battery packs, liberating the patient from reliance on cylinders.

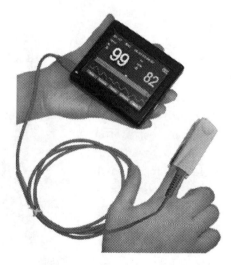

PULSE OXIMETER

For patients on long-term oxygen therapy, arterial oxygen measurements used to be mandatory for assessing changes in clinical status and to facilitate changes in the oxygen prescription. An arterial puncture to obtain blood for gas analysis yields very accurate results but gives only a snap-shot of what the clinical status was at the time of the arterial puncture. The blood, of course, has to be taken to a laboratory to be analysed. Pulse oximeters, on the other hand, are non-invasive and give direct measures of oxygen saturation, and the results are both immediate—in real time—and continuous. Home overnight pulse oximetry is useful to evaluate oxygen desaturation in patients with COPD during sleep. They are lightweight and portable, have memory and good battery life. Some models have become quite affordable.

In summary, supplemental oxygen therapy in patients with hypoxemia improves oxygen saturation levels, allows patients with COPD to maintain their mobility and increases their participation in the activities of daily living, such as cooking, shopping and exercising. There are, however, cautions to be observed:

1. Beware of having the oxygen flow too high, as this can cause accumulation of carbon dioxide (CO_2).
2. Do not smoke near oxygen.
3. If you plan to travel with oxygen, remember that your own oxygen cannot, in many parts of the world, be brought onto a flight. Alert the airline two weeks before travel begins, and request oxygen during the flight. Bring your own nasal cannula; airlines have only masks. Bring your oxygen prescription. The latest news on the subject of flying with oxygen is that the US Department of Transportation

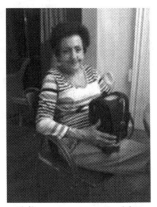

Airline passenger awaiting flight with portable oxygen concentrator[2].
Note nasal prongs.

---

[2]   Permission granted by patient, Mrs. G. Chasson, September, 2013

(DOT) ruled that air carriers conducting passenger capacity of more than 19 seats, must allow travellers with a disability to use an approved Portable Oxygen Concentrator (POC) on all flights.

4. Get a flu shot every year and request a pneumonia vaccination if you have not previously had one.

Surgery

As emphysema progresses, the walls of the air sacks, or alveoli, become more and more stretched, especially at the top of the lungs where alveoli are almost always larger than at the bottom of the lungs. Gradually, the stretching of the alveoli makes their walls longer and thinner. When that happens, the alveoli get so large and their walls so thin and fragile that they actually burst. Eventually they form one or more enormous air-containing spaces, like big balloons now uselessly occupying the top of the lung and even compressing what remains of "good" lung below. These big, useless air spaces are known as bullae, and when several of them have formed, the condition is known as bullous emphysema. Needless to say, the big bullous alveoli contribute nothing to respiration and result in increased shortness of breath, severe chest tightness, and increased breathing efforts to try to compensate for the upper parts of the lungs having been rendered useless. Sometimes the bullae rupture causing pneumothorax. In this complication, air escapes into the space between the lung and chest wall, further compressing the lung and causing intense pain.

Pneumothorax in a patient with COPD is an acute emergency. The air has to be drained from the pleural space before it not only compresses the underlying lung but also pushes down on the heart; this is a life-threatening situation demanding surgical intervention.

In some patients, elective rather than emergency surgery may be indicated to remove the bullae before disaster strikes.

Removing bullae (bullectomy) has a mortality rate variously reported as somewhere between 0-22percent, with some patients, probably about a third, maintaining the benefit of improved symptoms and blood oxygen for up to five years. The ideal candidate for surgery is one who has quit smoking and, despite medical therapy, has rapidly progressing shortness of breath. In some patients without obvious bullae detectable on computed tomography (CT) scanning, surgically removing the upper sections of lung with the large alveoli (lung reduction surgery) has been shown to produce short-term improvements in lung function, exercise tolerance, shortness of breath and quality of life. There is currently a strong perception that lung reduction surgery may also lead to long-term survival, but the statistical proof is not formally established yet. If it is, lung reduction surgery will join smoking cessation and supplemental long-term oxygen therapy as life-prolonging therapies for patients with COPD. The ideal candidate would be under the age of 75, with a clinical picture of emphysema, who has not smoked for at least six months, has severe shortness of breath, is maximally treated, including pulmonary rehabilitation, and is taking less than 20mg of prednisone a day.

Finally, there is lung transplantation. Three procedures are on offer: heart-lung, double lung and single lung transplant, the choice being determined to a large extent by the age of the patient. Heart-lung transplants are suitable for patients who are in their 50s or younger, and single lung transplants are suitable for the older patients. Timing is everything; transplantation should ideally not be performed when the patient is too ill. Fungal or tuberculosis infections of the lungs are relative contraindications, and the procedure should not be contemplated when there is underlying malignancy or musculoskeletal disease that inhibits chest wall movement. With careful patient selection, survival rates are as high as 80% at one year and 43% at five years. It is still not certain whether transplantation confers a survival advantage over the natural history of COPD, and unfortunately the prevalence of graft rejection in the form of obliterative bronchiolitis is as high as 70% among survivors. Compared with patients having other cardiopulmonary diseases, patients with emphysema have the best survival outcomes.

Pulmonary rehabilitation

In a perfect health care system, every patient with COPD would be offered a 6-12 week hospital-based program of exercise training, breathing strategies, and bronchial clearing. In addition, important components of the program would be education and monitoring of compliance with prescribed medications, psychological profiling, and support and assistance with the activities of daily living.

Home-based rehabilitation would of course be cheaper and more cost-effective, while allowing patients to remain in their own environments, close to family. The problem with home-based programs is that they are limited to a large extent to respiratory muscle training. Aside from not having the psychological support and close monitoring, patients at home have to forego such services as breathing into a device that increases positive end-expiratory pressure, thereby holding the airways open at the end of a breath to assist removal of bronchial secretions. Nonetheless, there is a growing amount of literature advocating home-based rehabilitation as a useful adjunct to COPD management.

The core component of a COPD rehabilitation regimen is education. Patients learn how to prevent acute relapses and to start early treatment of respiratory exacerbations, as well as receive useful tips on breathing strategies and how to clear their airways of secretions. The health care workers use postural drainage, percussion, positive pressure masks and assisted coughing, all directed to clearing the airways and unblocking bronchi that have become clogged with the inflammatory exudate that characterizes COPD and tortures those who suffer from it. These manoeuvres alone are responsible for much of the demonstrated, proven success of pulmonary rehabilitation.

In addition to the activities directed to "airway toilet" and "clearing the lungs," the other main focus of rehabilitation is exercise. It is the best way to improve muscle performance, both of limbs and of the muscles of breathing—intercostal, diaphragm, abdominal and neck. Patients undergo at least 20 sessions of comprehensive treatment. If they do, the expected result is clinically significant improvements in shortness of breath, improved muscle strength and endurance. Furthermore, it has now been shown that a good rehabilitation program will reduce mortality during hospital admissions, and improve health-related quality of life in COPD patients. Best of all, aside from being highly effective, rehabilitation is safe.

CHAPTER 8

Treatment of COPD: Pharmacological Therapy

Throughout the Asia-Pacific region—in Australia, China, India, Indonesia, Japan, Malaysia, Philippines, South Korea, Singapore and Taiwan—there are National Treatment Guidelines for COPD, which differ to some extent from country to country but which represent their method of choice. In addition to the individualized national guidelines adopted in these countries, the GOLD (Global Initiative for Chronic Lung Disease) guidelines are available and are followed in Hong Kong.

Generally, pulmonologists diagnose and treat COPD, but in Australia for instance, these activities, as in the US and many European countries, are taken over by allergists. In Australasia and Hong Kong, in addition to pulmonologists, COPD is frequently diagnosed and treated by family practitioners.

There are two essentially different phases of COPD treatment: Stable COPD and Acute Exacerbations.

The key points for pharmacological treatment of stable COPD according to the GOLD guidelines are reducing symptoms, reducing the frequency and severity of exacerbations, and improving health status and exercise tolerance. As a basic principle, long-term monotherapy with an oral or inhaled bronchodilator is not recommended for COPD or, for that matter, asthma.

1. Long-acting beta$_2$-agonists and long-acting anticholinergics are preferred over short-acting formulations.
2. Based on efficacy and side effects, inhaled bronchodilators are preferred over oral bronchodilators.
3. Long-term treatment with inhaled corticosteroids added to long-acting bronchodilators is recommended for patients at high risk of exacerbations.
4. A phosphodiesterase-4 inhibitor added to the above regimen is useful for reducing exacerbations, especially in patients with FEV$_1$ below 50%.
5. Influenza vaccines reduce risk of serious illness in patients with COPD.
6. Antibiotics should only be used for treating acute exacerbations.

The pharmacological treatment of acute exacerbations differs in key respects from the treatment of patients with stable COPD. During acute exacerbations, the worsening of respiratory symptoms far exceeds the normal day-to-day fluctuations that many patients experience. Bearing in mind that acute exacerbations are potentially life threatening and are most commonly precipitated by respiratory infections, the key points of drug treatment are the following:

1. Short-acting beta$_2$-agonists, preferably combined with short-acting anticholinergics, are the preferred bronchodilators for acute exacerbations.
2. Systemic (rather than inhaled) corticosteroids shorten recovery time and reduce the risk of early relapse.

3. Antibiotics are usually indicated and may help to reduce the length of hospital stays.

Recent trends in COPD care

1. The FDA does not recommend monotherapy treatment in obstructive pulmonary disease, i.e., asthma as well as COPD. Single agent long-acting beta$_2$-agonists such as salmeterol and formoterol, which do not contain a corticosteroid, will become less in demand, notwithstanding their proven efficacy and safety in clinical trials. These agents should in future be used in combination with controller medications—inhaled corticosteroids.

2. Inhalers that contain chlorofluorocarbons (CFCs), which are known to cause environmental damage, will be phased out. After the official phase-out date, products that contain CFCs cannot be made, dispensed or sold.

3. The selective, orally administered, long-acting inhibitor of the enzyme PDE-4, roflumilast, has been approved for patients with severe COPD. The drug is important because it is the first non-steroidal, oral, anti-inflammatory medication for COPD.

4. The best available, first-in-class combination of an inhaled corticosteroid and long-acting beta$_2$-agonist, containing fluticasone and salmeterol, is Seretide. The fixed dose combination, available as a dry powder in several doses, prevents inflammation and relaxes muscles in the airways to improve breathing. Hardly surprisingly, Seretide has become a blockbuster with revenues in excess of US$8 billion a year.

5. The gold-standard anticholinergic drug for COPD is Spiriva (tiotropium bromide). Indeed, it is at present the only long-acting anticholinergic on the market. Spiriva has met an important need for a non-adrenergic

bronchodilator that had specific efficacy for COPD rather than asthma, and sales are growing at a compound annual growth rate of over 18%. Its sales growth is expected to continue as the FDA has recently approved the additional indication of reductions of exacerbations in patients with COPD. The success of Spiriva will likely continue at least until competition from once daily, long-acting muscarinic receptor antagonists arrives to challenge its market position.

COPD therapy; the Asia problem

1. Have the drugs in the guidelines been approved everywhere?

There is considerable variation among Asian countries concerning drug approvals. Take, for example, the approved COPD therapies for first-line treatment. Whereas in Japan, long and short-acting beta$_2$-agonists, long and short-acting muscarinic receptor antagonists, inhaled corticosteroids and roflumilast are available for first-line treatment, but in Taiwan, only long-acting beta$_2$-agonists are approved. Hong Kong still recommends theophylline. By stark contrast, in South Korea, triple therapy with inhaled steroids, long-acting beta$_2$-agonists and long-acting muscarinic antagonists is the first-step regimen of choice. Asia is very diverse in terms of recommended treatment.

2. Are the approved drugs reimbursed?

It is one thing to have drugs available and recommended; it is quite another matter as to whether their purchase is reimbursed. At the present time, roflumilast is not reimbursed in any Asian country, whereas it is in most European countries. In India, there is absolutely no reimbursement for any COPD drug. Aside from roflumilast, all classes of COPD drugs are reimbursed in Australia, China, Hong Kong, Japan, Malaysia, and the Philippines, but in Taiwan, neither short- nor long-acting muscarinic antagonists are reimbursed. Asia is thus very diverse in terms of affordability of drugs.

3. What is the level of awareness of COPD in Asia?

Recently the Canadian Lung Association along with medical experts from the Canadian Thoracic Society issued a National Report Card on COPD, recognising the alarming increase in mortality. The main messages were that there was a shockingly low level of awareness and the disease was being managed poorly. While 98% of Canadians had awareness of breast cancer, HIV/AIDS and Alzheimer's disease, only 17% had any awareness of the term COPD. Canada has remarkably little diversity and only two official languages. A single federal government democratically rules the entire country, and its economy is one of the largest in the world. It ranks among the highest in international measurements of education, government transparency, civil liberties, quality of life and economic freedoms. Yet 83% of Canadians, it appears, have never heard of COPD.

If a country like Canada, where health care is free for everyone at the point of use, where services are also available from private providers, and where the government assures the quality of care through federal standards, one must surmise that in a diverse region such as Asia, it will be worse and complicated by the triple threat of smoking, pollution and haze. One can make a persuasive case for an epidemiological research study of COPD awareness across Asia. Such a study would likely be a complex one in the developing countries, where the prevalence of tuberculosis is so high that smokers with chronic cough might well have complex lung pathology with co-morbidities. Such patients, if fortunate enough to be correctly diagnosed and treated are, of course ineligible for either inhaled or systemic corticosteroids or to be recruited in clinical trials of immune modulating new therapies for COPD.

In Asia, with its well-recognized ethnic, economic, educational and social diversity, there is a lack of consistency even in the definition of COPD. Hence, in attempting to evaluate COPD epidemiology across Asia, using medical records and death certificates makes for scant and unreliable data. Throughout the world, with the exception of smoking cessation, factors in the development and manifestations of COPD have not received the attention of scientists or experts in health care delivery warranted by the public health importance of COPD. Awareness and subsequent effective management can be achieved only by a team approach that includes multiple disciplines. The initiatives of the GOLD programme will eventually raise global awareness of COPD. If these initiatives can be incorporated into Asian countries, the result will surely be a reduction of the burden of COPD in that part of the world where COPD is at its worst, and growing fastest.

The first challenge is to promote behavioural changes among healthcare professionals. The objective here is to translate research findings into clinical practise and public heath policies. The Cochrane Group, an international not-for-profit organisation preparing, maintaining and promoting the accessibility of systematic reviews of the effects of health care, has shown that passive dissemination of information by publication of consensus conferences in professional journals and the mailing of educational materials are ineffective in altering practices. Computerised decision support systems help to improve performances in decisions on drug dosages, preventative care and clinical management. Computerised systems have failed so far, however, to improve performance in the all-important area of diagnosing COPD.

The next challenge is to raise awareness in patients and their families through outreach programmes. For COPD we could do worse than follow the examples set by the U.S. National Heart, Lung and Blood Institute (NHLBI) and National Institutes of Health (NIH) in their work on hypertension, obesity and cholesterol. The NHLBI programmes are conducted through coordinating committees that have representatives from government agencies, medical and health care organizations and patient groups. In the case of asthma, for example, it has become clear that good scientific information and a network of partner organizations disseminating information can improve patient care. For COPD in Asia, what is needed is to follow these examples by establishing coalition groups to work at the community level to raise awareness of COPD and to improve diagnosis and care. Patient awareness is improved by the coordinated activities of local media, local thought leaders, and identification of target audiences, their demographics and their behaviours. The means of communication should ideally involve television, videos, radio, print media and support materials targeted to local news media outlets.

The GOLD programme has prepared a workshop report entitled "Global Strategy for Diagnosis, Management and Prevention of COPD," which has been widely circulated in multiple languages and which is updated every year. Every year GOLD sponsors a world COPD day with the theme of "Raising Awareness of COPD" in dozens of countries. They develop interactive programmes that directly engage audiences with health fairs conducted by local doctors. Public awareness is stimulated by questionnaires of the symptoms of COPD in local newspapers, magazines, and posters in subways and buses as well as in doctors' offices.

Much more needs to be done. In Japan, the Ministry of Health and Welfare in 1996 reported that the prevalence of COPD was 0.3% (i.e. almost non-existent)! Most formal studies since then have confirmed the more likely figure of between 8.6 and 10.9%, depending on the diagnostic criteria employed. The Ministry also claimed that the number of cases of COPD in patients over the age of 40 yrs. was only 0.2 million. Japanese physicians in Japan do not diagnose COPD in 90% of their patients who are known to have COPD by independent evaluation.

More work on COPD is also needed in China. If one takes the accepted criteria for diagnosis, an FEV_1 of less than 70% of vital capacity in smokers with chronic cough, in mainland China and Hong Kong, between 14.6 and 17% likely have COPD. Such is the level of under-diagnosis and lack of awareness that only 2.7% of these types of patients were actually diagnosed with COPD. The best estimate is that only one third of patients in China with clear lung function evidence of COPD had, in a recent study, been diagnosed with chronic bronchitis, emphysema or COPD. Furthermore, only one third of patients in hospitals have ever been tested for lung function. Education of health care professionals to use spirometry to evaluate patients, especially smokers, at high risk of developing COPD is desperately needed. The prevalence of COPD will continue to rise. Strategies to increase awareness in doctors and patients are desperately needed, as are plans to reduce tobacco consumption, air pollution, biomass fuels and occupational dusts.

CHAPTER 9

COPD Research:
Drugs in the Pipeline

A simple, web-based search into research in COPD generates approximately 12 million links. Among them, there is fascinating and indeed encouraging reading. Research has uncovered a wealth of information on the causes of COPD as well as ways in which the disease can and should be prevented and treated. Yet, many more unanswered questions remain: What is the role of genetic factors in lung damage? Why do all smokers develop airway inflammation, yet only 15% develop full-blown COPD? Can cost-effective, self-managed physical activity help patients improve their overall function? Does altering the physical properties and viscosity of mucous lessen damage to the airways? What role do bacteria and toxins in the body play in the development of COPD? These important questions receive the support of prestigious organizations like the NHLBI, but regrettably, progress has been slow in the development of new therapies that will, by tackling the destructive inflammatory process of COPD, prevent disease progression and mortality.

The current body of research information in the literature has focused very successfully on the pathogenesis of cigarette smoke, the protease/anti-protease balance, and increasingly on the epidemiology of COPD prevalence. In this latter respect, there is a yawning gap in our knowledge in Asia, but the tide is turning as the consequences of the gap in awareness are becoming more widely recognized.

What else needs to be done? At this stage, no treatments effectively suppress chronic inflammation in the lungs of COPD patients, and until such drugs are developed, we will continue to fail to prevent disease progression. Although the current tranche of mediator antagonists have so far been disappointing, the horizon is bright, as several new therapeutic targets have been identified and are being chased down. The main challenges are to find anti-inflammatory treatments that are safe and effective when administered orally and to see if corticosteroid resistance can be overcome.

Tackling airway inflammation

The advent of broncho-alveolar lavage as a simple method for harvesting inflammatory immune-effector cells from the lungs has greatly increased our appreciation of the cell types and numbers that characterize COPD as distinct from other conditions such as asthma and interstitial lung diseases. The knowledge does not seem, however, to have bridged some pressing gaps in our understanding of the specific role of inflammation in COPD. We still do not know why inflammation characteristic of COPD is seen in smokers who have not developed airways obstruction. We do not know why the inflammation persists long after a smoker quits. We remain puzzled as to why there is such a large overlap between the immune-effector cells harvested in patients with asthma and those with established COPD. Why, for example, do corticosteroids prevent and indeed reverse the inflammatory process in patients with asthma but fail to prevent progression in COPD? We do not even know whether the mucous hyper-secretion in COPD is partly responsible for worsening of COPD or just an annoying, unpleasant, distasteful symptom. Last but not least, why are the increased numbers of neutrophils and lymphocytes in lungs of patients with COPD lower than those found in other inflammatory lung conditions that do not destroy the lungs with the same devastating virulence?

The US Department of Health and Human Services and National Institutes of Health, at a workshop concerning future research directions for COPD, strongly urged the recruitment of more researchers with even further cooperation between universities and the pharmaceutical industry than already exists. The workshop prioritized further efforts to understand the pathology of COPD, particularly with regard to small airways, as a pressing need before new drug targets can be identified. The workshop recommended characterization of lung tissue correlated with clinical data using advanced methods of immunology, viral and microbial detection, molecular histopathology, microarray profiling of gene expression and proteomic analysis.

It identified the problem of a lack of readily measurable biomarkers that correlate with disease severity or outcome. It highlighted our gaps in knowledge in the inflammatory process, such that corticosteroids fail to slow down the decline in FEV_1. It urged family-based studies of genome-wide screening by linkage analysis of affected sibling pairs. It encouraged the use of animal models to test, for example, lung development and alveolar regeneration, especially in the late foetal and postnatal periods.

Chemokine receptor antagonists

Stopping the bad cells from swimming into the airways

Several new therapeutic targets have already been identified. One of the most encouraging is the research into CXCR2 antagonists that block pulmonary neutrophil and monocyte recruitment.

CXC chemokine receptors are membrane proteins that bind to cytokines of the CXC family. Chemokines are signalling proteins that are secreted by cells and are responsible for chemotaxis. Chemotaxis is the phenomenon whereby cells and bacteria move around according to certain chemicals in their environment. A simple example would be how bacteria swim towards the highest concentration of food molecules, or how a sperm swims towards an egg for fertilization. In the lung, interference with CXCR2 receptor function should theoretically inhibit pulmonary damage induced by neutrophils, mucous cell hyperplasia and scar tissue deposition caused by lung injury. After all, as Professor Peter Barnes, Head of Respiratory Medicine at Imperial College, London, has shown, the enzymatic and oxidative products from neutrophils, macrophages and lymphocytes are thought to cause the majority of the tissue degradation and destruction of lung tissue in emphysema. Initial reports from Schering-Plough Research Institute suggest that their small molecule CXCR2 antagonists, which block the chemotaxis of leukocytes, are now well advanced in clinical trials and hold considerable promise.

Phosphodiesterase-4 inhibitors

Broad-spectrum anti-inflammatory drugs

The phosphodiesterases are enzymes that catalyse the splitting of the phosphate linkage of nucleotide strands such as DNA and RNA. Inhibitors of the phosphodiesterases can be used as drugs, one of which, used to treat erectile dysfunction, is quite well known.

A nucleotide is a compound that has three important components: an aromatic base containing nitrogen, a sugar that is either ribose or deoxyribose and a phosphate group. DNA and RNA are long strands of nucleotides. Phosphate bonds form cyclic nucleotides. In every cell there are two types of cyclic nucleotides, cyclic AMP and cyclic GMP, which are known as the secondary messengers. For example, if a first signal comes from outside a cell by the binding of a hormone or neurotransmitter, an increase in cyclic AMP or cyclic GMP is triggered, and this greatly amplifies the magnitude of the original signal. So where do phosphodiesterases fit in? Phosphodiesterases degrade the cyclic nucleotides by splitting the phosphate bonds that keep the cyclic nucleotides cyclic.

There are many different types of phosphodiesterase; Viagra, Cialis and Levitra, for example, act through family five of the phosphodiesterases. Family three inhibitors are used in the treatment of heart failure.

Many compounds non-selectively inhibit some of the phosphodiesterases, the most ubiquitous being caffeine, classified as a minor stimulant—minor in comparison with other non-selective inhibitors that have been used in the past as asthma and COPD treatments, such as aminophylline and theobromine. Theophylline was for many years used to treat obstructive pulmonary disease, as it caused bronchodilation by inhibiting cyclic nucleotide phosphodiesterase (PDE), which inactivates cyclic AMP. By inhibiting PDE, theophylline increases cyclic AMP, suppressing inflammation and relaxing airway smooth muscle. There are now known to be many, many PDEs, each with differing activities, substrate preferences and tissue distributions.

The possibility exists to inhibit selectively only the enzymes in the tissues of interest, the interest here being the immune cells (macrophages, eosinophils and neutrophils) in the air-passages of the lungs. Inhibiting PDE-4 in these cells leads to increased cyclic AMP levels, thereby decreasing the quantity of the cellular component, i.e. down-regulating the inflammatory response. As PDE-4 is also expressed in airway smooth muscle, PDE-4 inhibitors relax these muscles. It is thus not surprising that selective PDE-4 inhibitors are the focus of much research activity for treating COPD.

Various PDE-4 inhibitors in medical practice have been shown to have anti-inflammatory effects in animal models and in patients with COPD. The latest of these medicines, roflumilast, has been shown to lead to significant reductions in exacerbations in patients with severe and very severe COPD. The patients who benefitted most were those with predominant chronic bronchitis rather than emphysema. Especially benefited were those concurrently taking concomitant inhaled corticosteroids. In general, clinical trials show modest but significant increases in lung function test results over placebo, improvements in quality of life scores and reduced numbers of exacerbations in the most severely affected patients. Both roflumilast and cilomilast reduce the number of inflammatory cells recruited into the airways and reduce the levels of biochemical markers of inflammation, such as interleukin-8 and neutrophil elastase.

Unfortunately, there is a drawback to the use of phosphodiesterase inhibitors. Since the days of theophylline, unwanted effects such as nausea, headache and diarrhoea have notoriously limited their use. As with their predecessors, studies with roflumilast and cilomilast have also shown some dose-limiting side effects such as diarrhoea, emesis and headache, but fortunately, none of the unwanted cardiovascular liabilities of older, non-selective drugs used in the past.

The most encouraging aspect of roflumilast from the point of view of patients and their prescribing physicians is that not only is it an orally administered selective phosphodiesterase-4 (PDE4) enzyme inhibitor, but it is also a once-a-day tablet. Roflumilast is the first drug in a new class of treatment for severe COPD, but it almost certainly will not be the last. It is the first oral anti-inflammatory treatment specifically developed for COPD patients.

The Global Initiative for Chronic Obstructive Lung Disease (GOLD) has included roflumilast (Daxas®) as a new treatment option in its COPD management guidelines.

Mitogen-activated protein kinases

Pulmonary shock absorbers

When phenomena such as inflammation, oxidative molecules, ultra-violet radiation and cytokines stress the lungs, a special group of proteins becomes activated. These proteins are known as the p38 subgroup of mitogen-activated protein kinases (MAPKs). Researchers such as Kian Fan Chung from the National Heart and Lung Institute, London, England, have shown that activation of the p38 pathway is involved in the pathogenesis of COPD. It follows therefore that this protein may be a suitable pharmacological target for therapeutic intervention, especially since the MAPKs in airway epithelial cells are known to be activated when exposed to cigarette smoke.

The MAPK family members include at least three distinct stress-activated protein kinase pathways: p38, c-Jun N-terminal kinase (JNK), and an extra-cellular regulating kinase (ERK). Although all three MAPKs interact in cellular processes, it is the p38 pathway that responds to environmental stresses. Currently, many researchers are focusing their attention on the development of small molecules aimed at inhibiting p38, and some of these molecules are now undergoing clinical trials.

The main reason for the intense interest in these studies is that particularly in COPD and to an extent in asthma, there is an unmet need known as steroid resistance. Some so-called refractory patients either fail to respond or respond poorly to existing anti-inflammatory treatments such as corticosteroids. It is hoped that the inhibition of activated protein kinases might eventually be useful in tackling steroid resistance.

There have already been some studies of p38 MAPK inhibitors in rheumatoid arthritis, other autoimmune diseases and insulin resistance in diabetes, but it appears that the first generation of molecules had unwanted effects on liver function. The second generation of drug candidates appears very promising, and there are many reasons for some confidence in a positive outcome in chronic airways disease. Activated p38 MAPK facilitates the movement of neutrophils and eosinophils into the lungs. MAPK releases pro-inflammatory cytokines from airway smooth muscle and participates in T-cell activation. The MAPKs cause airway wall remodelling and mucous cell hyperplasia, and they induce corticosteroid insensitivity.

Initial study results are encouraging, indeed. Research scientists at AstraZeneca (Ratcliffe and Dougal) compared the ability of a PDE-4 inhibitor, an inhaled steroid and a p38 mitogen-activated protein kinase inhibitor on the release of various inflammatory mediators from COPD lung transplant tissue. Whereas the effects of the PDE-4 inhibitor and the steroid budesonide were variable at best, treatment with the experimental p38 inhibitor (BIRB-796) inhibited TNF-alpha release from all specimens, including those that had responded poorly to steroids. These results suggest that a p38 inhibitor may in the future provide advantages over existing anti-inflammatory treatments for COPD, either as an add-on to existing therapy or to treat patients who respond poorly to steroids.

Increasing histone deacetylase-2 (HDAC2) activity

A change of target

What are histones? Histones are the proteins responsible for DNA storage. Our cells contain 23 pairs of chromosomes, giving a total of 46 in each and every cell. The human genome project has revealed that we have approximately 25,000 protein-coding genes. As only about 1.5% of the genome actually code for proteins, the rest of the genes are non-coding and are known as "junk DNA." At any one time, each of our cells is therefore using only a small proportion of its DNA, and the rest is stored safely out of reach. DNA storage is the job of the histone proteins. In the nucleus, DNA is wound around histones to form nucleosomes, which form part of the cell known as chromatin.

The behaviour of histones is controlled by the interplay of two enzymes: acetyl transferase and deacetylase. These two enzymes are prime targets for cancer chemotherapy. When drugs inhibit deacetylase, a cancer cell can be changed from one that grows without limit to a differentiated cell that does not multiply at all. It gets even more interesting; drugs that stimulate acetylation induce an arrest of the cell cycle, stopping all further growth and inducing "cell suicide" or, perhaps more correctly, programmed death of tumour cells.

Accordingly, there has been considerable effort to develop histone deacetylase inhibitors (HDIs) for the treatment of cancer. One of the best known of these medications is Vorinostat for the treatment of patients with skin involvement from T-cell lymphoma. The HDIs are also under investigation for HIV treatment and as sensitizers for cytotoxic chemotherapy and radiotherapy.

Histone deacetylase inhibitors (HDIs) have a long history of use in psychiatry as mood stabilizers and in neurology for the treatment of epilepsy, valproic acid being one of the better known anti-epilepsy drugs in wide-spread use.

The current interest for our purposes is that HDAC is a key molecule in the repression of production of inflammatory cytokines in COPD. The total amount of HDAC activity is decreased in the lung tissue, bronchial walls and alveolar macrophage cells of patients with COPD compared with age-matched smokers who do not have COPD. This remarkable observation is all the more interesting because the researchers did not find a reduction of HDAC activity in the lungs of patients with cystic fibrosis or pneumonia. Furthermore, a positive correlation was seen between HDAC activity and disease severity. These findings indicate that there are likely therapeutic implications, as the reductions in HDAC activity appear to be reversible. The phosphodiesterase inhibitor—the bronchodilator drug theophylline, for example—activates HDAC. HDAC activity plays an important part in mediating the anti-inflammatory effects of corticosteroids in COPD patients. When HDAC activity is diminished or lost, the result will likely be a loss of therapeutic activity of the steroids (steroid resistance), as well as an increase in the expression of inflammatory cytokines such as IL-8, and inevitably an increase in disease activity. A cause for concern is that non-selective suppression of HDAC activity by anti-cancer drugs may well have a detrimental effect in patients with COPD.

New drugs for COPD

Good news or bad news?

Chronic bronchitis and emphysema are the diseases that comprise COPD. Although COPD is one of the most prevalent diseases in the world, suffered by literally hundreds of millions of people, therapeutic options for the treatment of COPD are limited, in marked contrast to asthma. There is a great unmet need in the market. The inhaled medication tiotropium bromide (Spiriva) approved for the treatment of COPD in 2004 and for reduction of COPD exacerbations as recently as 2009, was the first specific drug for COPD approved by the FDA. The combination drug Advair (fluticasone/salmeterol) which is used for COPD, was initially approved for asthma, not specifically for COPD. Similarly Symbicort, the combination of budesonide/formoterol, which is now used for COPD, was originally approved for treatment of asthma.

Aside from roflumilast, the orally administered selective phosphodiesterase-4 (PDE4) enzyme inhibitor, once-a-day tablet, which is now approved (but not in Asian markets yet) and recommended by GOLD guidelines, novel pipeline therapies for treatment of COPD are sparse. Until the big break-through arrives, the best we can hope for is more long acting, dual-action bronchodilator/steroid combinations.

CHAPTER 10

COPD Action Plans:
Surely There is More We Can Do

According to the Global Risks Report at the World Economic Forum in 2011, chronic diseases are a global risk equal in cost to the global financial crisis that began in 2008. Without urgent collective action, the effects of these risks will be felt for years to come. COPD is not a smoker's cough; it is a life-threatening lung disease.

The European COPD Coalition has issued a call to action to be taken at the European national and local levels to tackle the epidemic of COPD. Specifically, the Coalition has implored the supporting member states to recognize the political importance of acting on COPD, to facilitate appropriate and effective actions and to ensure the EU protects public health. Coalition members want strong messages against smoking, implementation of the recommendations made by the WHO's Convention on Tobacco Control, increased financing of public health campaigns on risk factors and promotion of early screening and diagnosis of people at risk.

The European COPD Coalition has the strong support of the Canadian Thoracic Society and Lung Association, who have issued a National Report Card on COPD, the largest and most in-depth research study ever completed on COPD in Canada. Canadian men and women are dying from COPD at a startling rate. Of the leading causes of death, COPD is the only one with an increasing mortality. Hospitalization rates are also high and climbing.

Awareness of the disease, its symptoms and its risk factors is very low compared to other leading causes of death, even among those most at risk. The goal of the Report Card was to highlight the strengths and gaps in COPD prevention and management and to put the disease on the national and provincial healthcare agendas. The bottom line: COPD needs to be on the agendas. The recommendations, of similar vein to those in Europe, set a standard that hopefully will find traction in the diverse region of Asia, where COPD has more potent risk factors, woeful lack of awareness, lack of compliance with treatment guidelines and comparative lack of drug availability and reimbursement. In summary, the Canadian recommendations are:

- Prioritize COPD in healthcare by developing a strategy across the country and allocate funding specifically for COPD.
- Implement public awareness and education initiatives about COPD risks, symptoms and treatments.
- Create pulmonary rehabilitation and fund rehab programs.
- Provide patient reimbursement for medications to reflect the treatment guidelines.
- Expand training of physicians for better awareness of GOLD and National guidelines and use of lung-function testing.
- Fund smoking prevention and cessation programs.

How should research funding be allocated?

Clearly, the public health measures outlined above are urgently needed. From the purely research point of view, scientists and physicians see challenges that, if met, are likely to yield untold rewards in terms of benefit to millions of patients as well as commercial opportunities to fund future research. The current areas of interest that are attracting cooperation between universities and the pharmaceutical industry are first of all to improve our knowledge regarding the pathology of COPD and secondly to discover disease-modifying drugs that stimulate regeneration of lung tissue.

1. Description of the COPD disease process

One of the biggest mysteries is what process is responsible for damage to the small airways. We know that in COPD, the small airways become inflamed, but we do not really know the cellular or chemical processes that take place and how the damage relates to clinical manifestations of the disease. Somehow, we need to do a better job of comparing lung structural, inflammatory and biochemical characteristics with clinical history of symptoms, lung-function status and the course of the disease. One approach might be to obtain surgical specimens from patients with suspected lung cancer and subject the tissue to immunology, viral and micro-array profiling of gene expression.

Another approach might be to discover measurable biomarkers and intermediate end-points that can be monitored and that would correlate with disease severity and outcome. Examples that are being explored are chemicals in the breath, sputum or blood that reflect lung inflammation, and detailed lung imaging studies by CT, MRI or PET in smokers with and without COPD.

Furthermore, what are the genetic factors that determine immune responsiveness? What genetic factors determine susceptibility to lung injury? These questions can be addressed only by studying multiple phenotypes. Different genes may be related to susceptibility, tendency to suffer exacerbations, rate of progression and whether smoking will lead to the patient's being a pink puffer or a blue bloater. Family studies are needed, with attention to screening by linkage analysis of affected sibling pairs.

There is a mystery surrounding the causes and consequences of acute exacerbations, usually attributed by patients and their physicians to simple respiratory tract infections. There must, however, be some explanation as to what environmental insults and immune responses underlie whom and when respiratory infections strike, as well as an explanation of the pathological process by which symptoms subsequently worsen after respiratory infections strike.

Is the production of mucous in patients with COPD a benefit or a risk? This, too, is not known! We need more research into the molecular and cellular mechanisms of excess mucous production.

2. New treatments

To date, and as noted earlier, there is no firm statistical proof that any of the remarkable drug therapies that improve symptoms and quality of life in patients with COPD actually increase survival. Only long-term oxygen therapy and smoking cessation, at the time of writing, have been proven to prolong life in patients with COPD. The situation will change, one might speculate, when scientists have learned how to stimulate alveolar regeneration. Disease-modifying therapies will likely come from animal studies of alveolar development, especially in the late foetal and post-natal periods. Research techniques will involve gene expression and proteomic analysis of the developing lung, regulation of expression of relevant genes and studies of how blood vessels in the lung develop and repair. According to an

NHLBI workshop on "Future Research Directions in COPD." the approach most likely to provide answers will be the study of lung development and repair in transgenic mice to see how toxins such as nicotine impair lung growth and to explore conditions in which alveolar regeneration can occur.

CHAPTER 11

Lung-function Testing in COPD: Is the FEV_1 Out-dated?

In obstructive pulmonary disease, the rate at which air can be blown out of the lungs is reduced due to narrowing of the airways. As one exhales forcibly, the airways become more and more compressed due to the positive pressure in the chest, squeezing the airways as the air is forced out. As the exhalation goes on, the flow of air gradually decreases, as anyone who has tried to blow out candles on a birthday cake can recognize. The extent of the airway narrowing is measured by calculating the ratio between the amount of air exhaled in the first second after starting to blow, in relation to the amount of air that can be exhaled if the

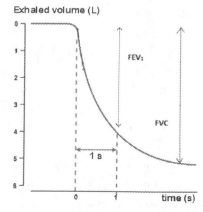

patient is given enough time to exhale maximally. The FEV_1 is the term used to describe the maximal amount of air that can be blown out in one second. The FVC (Forced Vital Capacity) is a measure of the amount of air that can be forcibly exhaled from the lungs after taking the deepest breath possible. Measuring FEV_1 and FVC is done by spirometry, (lung function testing) and can be performed simply in the physician's office or in a pulmonary function laboratory. The diagnosis of airways obstruction, or narrowing, is made when the FEV_1/FVC ratio is reduced below 80%.

Various authorities have slight differences in how spirometry should be interpreted. According to the National Institute for Clinical Excellence (NICE), the diagnosis of COPD is made when the FEV_1/FVC ratio is less than 70%. On the other hand, the Global Initiative for Obstructive Lung Disease (GOLD) states that the reduced level of FEV_1/FVC is acceptable for the diagnosis of COPD only if the ratio remains reduced after bronchodilator has been given. This is a fair point; in asthma the ratio is also reduced, but it will likely partially respond, or even be reversed, by inhaling a beta-2 agonist bronchodilator. Yet a third interpretation of FEV_1 is given by the European Respiratory Society (ERS), which compares the FEV_1 to normal, predicted values according to age, height, ethnicity and gender. Obstructive lung disease, the ERS says, can be diagnosed if the patient's FEV_1 is less than 88% of the predicted value for men or 89% for women.

Vital capacity as a measure of lung function has been with us since John Hutchinson invented the spirometer in 1842. The birth of the FEV_1 came much later when Robert Tiffeneau in Paris in 1947 and Edward Gaensler from Boston University in 1950, realized that measuring flow was of critical diagnostic importance in patients with lung disease and described the principles of measuring airflow.

Unarguably, lung function testing, specifically in the form of measuring FEV_1 and the FEV_1/FVC ratio, is an essential component of the diagnostic work-up for COPD. Furthermore, in some types of airways obstruction such as asthma, the FEV_1 is an appropriate marker of response to treatment. In asthma, by definition, the airway obstruction is reversible. In COPD, the airway obstruction, by definition, is not. How then can the repeated measurement of FEV_1 as a study endpoint in patients with COPD be a sensible means for assessing responses to therapy in clinical research projects?

Questioning the value of FEV_1 as an end-point for COPD drug trials

1. What does the FEV_1 actually measure?

The FEV_1 curve reflects first of all the elastic recoil of the lung. Take a big breath in, hold it and let go. The air that comes out in the first half-second or so is purely a result of lung elastic recoil. After the initial, upper part of the curve, the remainder of the FEV_1 reflects resistance to airflow in the large and medium-sized airways. Resistance to airflow in these segments of the lung is exactly what is reduced in asthma and is the target of anti-asthmatic drugs. Accordingly, whereas the FEV_1 is the accepted gold standard for both clinical management and efficacy outcome for asthma, there surely should be scepticism or doubt as to its relevance in COPD. COPD is a different kettle of fish from asthma. In COPD, the main burden of inflammatory pathology is in the small airways. The FEV_1 does not measure or reflect small airway narrowing, as the flow limitation in the small airways is not apparent until late in the maximum exhalation, after the one second time interval has passed. The hallmark of COPD is lung hyperinflation. The increased lung volumes that are seen in COPD arise from premature closure of small airways, resulting in gas trapping. The evaluation of new medicines for the treatment of patients with COPD should therefore include some assessment of lung volumes. The FEV_1 is not a measure of volume. It is a measure of flow. Indeed, it is a basic single unit of flow-volume as a function of time or litres/second. Unfortunately, the flow that is measured by the FEV_1 is not during the phase of a breath that is of interest in COPD. In COPD we need to assess flow rates towards the end of the breath, when small airways are progressively narrowing and eventually closing completely.

2. Is there a better test for measuring flow rate in small airways?

The spirometry test known as the flow/volume loop has several advantages over the FEV_1. First, instead of a single measure of flow, the flow/volume curve gives a continuous measure of flow throughout the breath; both while taking a maximum breath in and then while exhaling as hard and fast as possible, just like in the FEV_1 manoeuvre. The curve begins on the X-axis, or volume axis. At the start of the test, both flow and volume are zero, and then as exhalation starts, the curve rapidly climbs to a peak: the Peak Expiratory Flow. The Peak Expiratory Flow (PEF) then descends as the flow rate diminishes as more and more air is exhaled from the lungs. In a healthy subject, the loop will descend in a straight line from top (Peak Flow) to the bottom (Forced Vital Capacity or FVC). In patients with obstructive pulmonary disease

such as asthma and COPD, the down slope of the loop is no longer a straight line, but a concave curve. The air in the large airways can be exhaled without problem. The peak flow might well be normal but in COPD for example, the small airways are partially blocked so the air comes out from them slowly. The result is that when the breath is 50% finished, and then when there

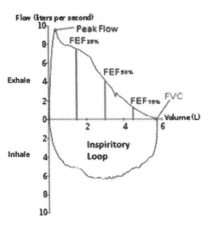

is only 25% of the breath left, flow will be markedly reduced. Accordingly, Forced Expiratory Flow at 50% of the curve ($FEF_{50\%}$) and Forced Expiratory Flow when three quarters through the breath ($FEF_{25\%}$) will be very reduced. These are findings in early COPD that would not be detected in the FEV_1 or FEV_1/FVC ratio.

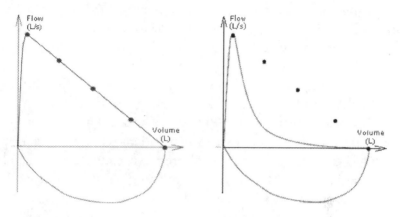

3. Does the FEV_1 correlate well with COPD outcome?

The Honolulu Heart Study showed clearly that the rate of decline in lung function over a six-year period was a significant predictor of mortality in men with COPD and that the association was stronger for smokers than non-smokers. In the Baltimore Longitudinal Study of Ageing, the rate of decline in lung function was an independent predictor of mortality for men from heart disease. The West Australian Busselton Study, which was conducted from 1969-1981, further showed the association between decline in FEV_1 and mortality, independent of risk factors for cardiovascular disease, cigarette smoking and the initial level of FEV_1.

In healthy non-smoking people, the FEV_1 declines at a rate of 15-30 ml/year between the ages of 25-50. After the age of 50 the decline speeds up and becomes 30-50 ml/year, the faster the decline, the greater mortality risk. COPD is a disease of rapidly declining FEV_1, and the principal factor associated with decline in FEV_1 is cigarette smoking. Smoking is not the only known risk factor for accelerated decline in lung function; others include asthma, childhood respiratory infections, occupational hazards, and, of course, pollution. While the FEV_1 is invaluable in epidemiological studies for diagnosing COPD and for following the steady decline in overall lung function, there is increasing evidence that it is a poor reflector of overall well being and response to therapy.

Nonetheless, the most widely accepted marker for COPD is the FEV_1, and it remains a key primary outcome required by regulatory authorities for COPD clinical trials. The justification for this requirement is unclear, when patient-reported outcomes such as health status, shortness of breath, exercise tolerance and exacerbations are of far greater interest to physicians. The FEV_1 is, in fact, only modestly associated with change in health status.

The non-scientist physician on learning that a clinical trial of a new drug for COPD resulted in an increase in FEV_1 could be excused for wondering if this is really possible in a disease in which FEV_1 **by definition** progressively declines over time, as it does even in healthy subjects. Does a claim of an increase in FEV_1 really mean that FEV_1 did not decline as much as the placebo control? Or does it mean that some of the patients actually had a component of asthma rather than 'pure' COPD. Scepticism about the sacred cow status of FEV_1 is reinforced on reading that bronchodilator drugs can improve lung mechanics in COPD patients despite little change in FEV_1 due to a decrease in hyperinflation of the lungs.

4. Proposal for a lung function test that reflects improvement in lung volume

The ratio of FEV_1 to FVC has long been the parameter-of-choice to define the presence of airflow limitation. The problem with FVC is that it is a measure of volume rather than flow rate and that it is heavily influenced by the duration of the expiratory time. When in elderly patients the lungs are slowly emptied during a maximal exhalation, the recorded FVC is influenced by the expiratory time. A simplified alternative to the FVC manoeuvre is the FEV_6, the volume of air that can be exhaled in six seconds. Several authors have proposed the FEV_6 as a surrogate for FVC in spirometry.

For the patient, the FEV_6 is less demanding than the FVC, particularly in the elderly. In patients with an obstructive disease, an FVC measure, which requires a prolonged period of urging the patient to "blow, blow, blow" for many seconds, leads to a period of coughing, occasional fainting, complaining, distress and unwillingness to complete the designated protocol of three technically satisfactory recordings. Accordingly, the FEV_6 is easier to obtain and therefore more reproducible than the FVC.

The hallmark of COPD is lung hyperinflation. The increased lung volumes that are seen in COPD arise from premature closure of small airways, resulting in gas trapping and a loss of lung elastic recoil. It seems reasonable to propose therefore that the evaluation of new medicines for treatment of patients with COPD should include some assessment of lung volume.

Lung hyperinflation changes the mechanical efficiency of the diaphragm, flattening out its normal curvature, rendering it more susceptible to fatigue. In order to maintain an adequate level of ventilation, the patient needs to make use of other muscles such as intercostal and the accessory muscles in the neck to move the upper ribs. It is not surprising that in patients with COPD, measures of lung volume and hyperinflation correlate well with shortness of breath.

What measures of lung volume would be most appropriate for evaluation in clinical drug trials for patients with COPD?

The most accurate, albeit complicated and technically demanding, would be measurements taken in a body plethysmograph. This technique gives accurate, precise measures of the residual volume trapped in the lung after a forced expiration (Residual Volume—RV) and the total amount of air in the lungs after a maximal breath in (Total Lung Capacity—TLC). The surrogate of these gold standard measurements is the FVC or forced vital capacity.

In designing a clinical trial many factors must be taken into consideration, such as the technical skills of the researcher, practicability, availability of equipment, technical support, patient cooperation and applicability to day-to-day practice.

Plethysmographic measures of lung volume require sophisticated techniques that are not always available in every pulmonary function laboratory. Even if available, equipment, calibration and standardization of techniques vary from one laboratory to another. Sadly, no matter how useful it would be to know the volume of trapped air, plethysmography has no place in a high volume, routine medical practice.

5. The FEV_6

In order to simplify the measurement of forced vital capacity, a more reproducible, physically less demanding alternative is proposed: the forced expired volume in six seconds.

The FEV_6 lends itself well to office spirometry. It is suitable for use by primary care practitioners, internists, nurse practitioners and GPs.

The Lung Health and Education Program (NLHEP) proposed the FEV_6 as a means of identifying the millions of people with undiagnosed COPD.

The FEV_6 can be used as a surrogate for the FVC.

Notwithstanding the conservatism in physicians and reluctance of regulatory authorities to accept wholeheartedly the FEV_6 in place of the FVC, it is an excellent epidemiological tool, and could be included, at least for now, as a secondary end-point when FVC is selected as the primary outcome in clinical research.

Finally, if a new treatment directed at improving small airway function is successful, gas trapping and residual volume will decrease. These highly satisfactory outcomes will almost certainly not be reflected in an increase in FEV_1, but they will most likely be seen as an improvement in FEV_6.

It is gratifying to see that in Asia, the FEV_6 has started to find a place in diagnosing COPD. Recognizing that the FEV_6 is more pleasant for the patient and more convenient for the tester than the FVC, investigators at the Philippines Heart Centre tested 597 Asian subjects and established the validity, sensitivity and specificity of FEV_1/FEV_6 in diagnosing moderate airways obstruction.

In addition, the PLATINO project, which was set up to study the prevalence of COPD in Latin American countries (Brazil, Chile, Mexico, Uruguay and Venezuela), has shown that the FEV_1/FEV_6 is a more robust and more reliable index in providing comparisons of COPD prevalence than the traditional (more variable) FEV_1/FVC.

Perhaps FEV_6, a simple measure that reflects lung volume rather than irreversible flow limitation, will find a secure and meaningful place as a primary efficacy end-point in community-based COPD treatment studies in the future.

COPD and Diabetes: Time Bombs and Gathering Storms

Early in the preparation of this book, it became apparent to the author that Asia was simultaneously facing two eerily similar epidemics, COPD and type 2 diabetes. However, colleagues tended to greet this observation with something between scepticism and a rolling of the eyes. It was not until a fortuitous meeting with the highly respected endocrinologist Professor Mark Cooper from Melbourne that it became obvious that the similarities were so striking that a formal comparison between the two diseases was worthy of documentation (Cooper ME and Rebuck AS. *J Diabetes*, Oct. 17, 2013).

Type 2 diabetes has reached epidemic proportions worldwide and represents a major threat to global health. Over the last 20 years, this problem has been particularly serious in the Asian region, most markedly in East Asia.

Like COPD, type 2 diabetes is a progressive condition whose cause is related to lifestyle and for which the objective of management is limited to slowing the inexorable course of the disease. Until recently type 2 diabetes has received only moderate priority in terms of research funding and has been subject to limited public awareness. Like COPD, type 2 diabetes was for many years considered to be a disease limited to the middle-aged and elderly. Both are now appearing in younger adults. Last but not least, it is now recognized that aside from lifestyle causes, in type 2 diabetes there is an interaction between nutrient intake and genetic factors, probably as a result of a range of epigenetic pathways.

Let us examine in further detail the similarities between Chronic Obstructive Pulmonary Disease and Type 2 Diabetes:

1. The burden of both type 2 diabetes and COPD has been underestimated for many years.
2. The prevalence of both disorders is rising rapidly, and both are now leading causes of death.
3. The objective of management of both diseases is limited to slowing progression. There is no cure for either and both are to a large extent avoidable.
4. The level of awareness of COPD and type 2 diabetes by the public and by physicians is generally poor, particularly in rural regions.
5. The major impact of both type 2 diabetes and COPD in the future will be in Asia.
6. Both disorders may be mitigated by life-style changes.
7. Research into COPD and type 2 diabetes has been underfunded, compared, for example, with cancer.
8. There are only limited resources for treatment of both disorders in developing countries.
9. The current estimate is that there are just over 300 million people in the world with COPD and just over 300 million people in the world with type 2 diabetes.

10. Both disorders were originally thought to be diseases of the elderly, but there are now increasing numbers of young people with type 2 diabetes and COPD.
11. There is an interaction between genetic and environmental factors in the pathogenesis and progression of both disorders.

There is little or no argument regarding the benefit of life-style changes to reduce body weight as a key component of type 2 diabetes management. People who lose weight are more likely to achieve partial or complete diabetes remission than those who do not. Similarly, the literature is replete with the proven benefit of smoking cessation in the management of COPD.

There is now convincing evidence that combining life-style changes with medication is more efficacious in slowing the progression of diabetes than medication alone—just like COPD.

In diabetes, there is a need for new, safe, more effective drugs that will not only produce sustained, meaningful improvements in laboratory tests (blood glucose) but that will also slow the loss of beta-cell function. Just as is the case with COPD, we need new drugs that will improve lung function and at the same time alter the inflammation-induced loss of lung elastic tissue.

In this book, COPD in Asia has been referred to as a gathering storm. Professor Cooper often describes diabetes as a ticking time bomb. We propose that lessons might be learned from a meeting of the minds across the two disciplines, each of which is facing a set of common challenges.

SOURCES

INTRODUCTION

1. Surprising Natural Lessons from Mount St. Helens. What have scientists learned from 30 years of research and rebirth in the blast zone? Scientific American. May 19, 2010.
2. Mount St. Helens Eruption: Facts & Information. Livescience. February 28, 2013.
3. Tilling, Robert I., Topinka, Lyn and Swanson Donald A. "Eruptions of Mount St. Helens: Past, Present and Future". *The Climactic Eruption of May 18, 1980*. U.S. Geological Survey. December 5, 2010.
4. Mount St. Helens Eruption. May 18, 1980. Angela Brown. About.com. Guide.

CHAPTER 1 BREATHING POISON

HAZE

1. Thomas F. Saarinen. Warning and Response to the Mount St. Helens Eruption. (SUNY Series in Environmental Public Policy). www.amazon.com
2. The Tucson Arizona Daily Star. 18 May. 1981.
3. Genesis: chapter 2, verse 7.

4. H. E. Taylor and F. E. Lichte. Chemical composition of Mount St. Helens volcanic ash. Geophysical Research Letters. Volume 7, issue 11, 1980.
5. Volcanic ash: effects and mitigation strategies. Volcanies. usgs.gov/ash/properties.html.
6. A.S. Buist, R.S. Bernstein, L.R. Johnson and W.M.Volmer. Evaluation of physical health effects due to volcanic hazards: human studies. Am. J. Public Health. 76(Suppl):66-75, March 1986.
7. Horwell, CJ, Baxter, PJ. The respiratory health hazards of volcanic ash: a review for volcanic ash mitigation. Bulletin of Volcanology. 69, 1-24, 2006.
8. Buist AS, McBurnie MA, Vollmer WM, Gillespie S, Burney P, Mannino DM, Menezes AM, Sullivan SD, Lee TA, Weiss KB, Jensen RL, Marks GB, Gulsvik A, Nizankowska-Mogilnicka E; BOLD Collaborative Research Group. Lancet. 380:806, 2012.
9. S. Buist. Expanding our knowledge of COPD. Lancet. 370; 733, 2007.
10. Smoke Engulfs Singapore. NASA Earth Observatory. 21 June. 2013.
11. J. He, B. Zielinska and R. Balasubramanian. Composition of semi-volatile organic compounds in the urban atmosphere of Singapore: influence of biomass burning. Atmos. Chem. Phys. Discuss. 10, 8415, 2010.
12. Haze in Singapore hits PSI all-time record. Yahoo news. 29 June, 2013.
13. Four times as many hotspots in Sumatra now. http://thestar. com
14. Cheam, J. Haze hits hazardous levels, Singapore and Indonesia at war of words. www.eco-business.com.
15. WWF renews calls for zero-burn policies to be enacted. Channel News Asia. 28 June, 2013.
16. General Health Advice during Haze. Ministry of Health Brunei, Darussalam. 27 June, 2013.

17. Pekanbaru's airport shut down due to thick haze. Antara News. 30 June. 2013.
18. Why Indonesia can only wait for rain as Riau burns and Singapore chokes. The Jakarta Globe. 21 June, 2013.
19. Eight Indonesians arrested as Singapore haze creeps back. Inside Investor. 27 June. 2013.
20. Haze shrouds Singapore and Malaysia. Online Wall Street Journal. 18 June, 2013.
21. The Singapore child is being suffocated. Goh Chok Tong. Channel News Asia. 21 June, 2013.
22. Foreign Minister to discuss Indonesian wildfire at ASEAN. National News Bureau of Thailand. 27 June, 2013.
23. Indoor Air Quality in Asian Countries. Sept. 2012. www.envirotech-online.com
24. Indoor Air Pollution: The Air I breathe. Asian Tribune. Volume 12; 498, 2013.
25. Indoor Air Pollution, Health and the Burden of Disease: cooking and heating with solid fuels. World Health Organization. www.who.int/indoorair.com
26. David Pennise and Kirk Smith. Biomass pollution basics. www.who.int/indoorair
27. Indoor air pollution and household energy. www.who.int/heli/risks/indoorair

AIR POLLUTION

1. C.A. Pope and D.W. Dockery. Air pollution and life expectancy in China and beyond. Proc. Natl. Acad. Sci. 110:12861, 2013.
2. Y. Chen, A. Eberstein, M. Greenstone and L. Hongbin. Evidence on the impact of sustained exposure to air pollution on life expectance from China's Huai River policy. Proc. Natl. Acad. Sci. July 8. 2013.
3. World Economic Forum Davos 2012: India at 125th position in Environmental Performance Index. Jan 25. 2012.

4. Pollution rise worsens South Asia's winter smog. www.bbc. co.uk/news

5. Iqbal Habib. Third International Conference on Bangladesh Environment. Dhaka University, Jan. 3-4, 2010.

6. Pollution kills 15,000 Bangladeshis each year. BAPA (Bangladesh Environmental Improvement Organization). American Society for Public Administration. www.patimes. org.

7. Pollution fears over Delhi smog. BBC NEWS, Delhi. Nov. 13. 2008.

8. The most polluted places on earth. CBS News. Jan. 8, 2010. www.cbsnews.com

9. Newly detected air pollutant mimics damaging effects of cigarette smoke. www.physorg.com

10. David Pennise and Kirk Smith. "Biomass Pollution Basics". www.who.int.com

11. Ambient Air Pollution: Health Hazards to Children. Committee on Environmental Health. Pediatrics. 114:1699, 2004.

12. Polluted Cities: The Air Children Breathe. World Health Organization. www.who.int/che/publications/airpollution.

13. Goss C.H., Newsom S.A, Schildcrout J.S., Sheppard L. and Kaufman J.D. Effect of ambient air pollution on pulmonary exacerbations and lung function in Cystic Fibrosis. American Journal of Respiratory and Critical Care Medicine. 169:816, 2004.

14. Zoidis J.D. The impact of air pollution on COPD. Decision makers in respiratory care. 1999. www.rtmagazine.com.

15. Laden F, Schwartz J, Speizer FE, et al. Reduction in fine particulate air pollution and mortality: extended follow-up of the Harvard Six Cities Study. Am J Respir Crit Care Med. 173:667, 2006.

16. Seinfeld J. and Spyros P. Atmospheric Chemistry and Physics: From Air Pollution to Climate Change. John Wiley and sons. 1998.

17. Upton J. Where is the worst air in the world? Medical examiner. 2013. www.slate.com/articles/health.
18. WHO survey Asian Pollution index. www.asianconversations.com
19. Southeast Asia's worst air pollution. Times of India. Sept. 3. 2013.
20. US doctors fight air pollution in Mongolia's capital. July 23.2013. www.asianscientist.com
21. Tyler Falk. World's worst air pollution in Iran and South Asia. www.smartplanet.com
22. Pollution causes 470,000 premature deaths in China every year—too high a price to pay for industrialization? www.rainbowbuilders.org/china
23. BC Lung Association 2005 report on the valuation of health impacts from air quality in the Lower Fraser Valley. www.bc.lung.ca
24. Kahn J. and Yardley J. "As China roars, Pollution Reaches Deadly Extremes." Aug 26, 2007. www.nytimes.com
25. China buried smog death finding. July 3. 2007 http://news.bbc.co.uk

SMOKING

1. www.biography.com/people/albert-einstein
2. Einstein: His Life and Universe by Walter Isaacson: Simon and Schuster, 2007.
3. Who was Albert Einstein? By Jess M. Brallier. Amazon.com
4. Tobacco: A Cultural History of How and Exotic Plant Seduced Civilization. Ian Gately: google.com.sg
5. Tobacco and Shamanism in South America. J. Wilbert. Yale University Press, 1987
6. Tobacco in History. J. Goodman. Routledge, 1993.
7. Likint F. *Tabak and Tabakrauch als aetiolischer Factor des Carcinoms.* (Tobacco and tobacco smoke as etiological factors for cancer). Krebsforsch Z: 30:349, 1929.

8. Proctor R. The Nazi War on Tobacco: Ideology, Evidence and Possible Cancer Consequences. Bulletin of the History of Medicine. 71:435, 1997.

9. Smith G.D. Lifestyle, health and health promotions in Nazi Germany. British Medical Journal.329:1424, 2004.

10. Bignon V. Smoking or trading? On cigarette money in post WW2 Germany. Economix. University of Paris. 2003.

11. Doll R., Hilly B.A. Smoking and carcinoma of the lung. Preliminary report. British Medical Journal. 2:739, 1950.

12. Doll R., Hilly B.A. The mortality of doctors in relation to their smoking habits; a preliminary report. British Medical Journal 1:1451, 1954.

13. United States Surgeon General's Advisory Committee on Smoking and Health. United States. Public Health Service. Office of the Surgeon General Public Health Service Publication No. 1103, 1964.

14. Rock VJ., Malarcher A., Kahende JW. et al. Cigarette smoking among adults. United States Centers for disease control and prevention. www.cdc.gov. 2006.

15. WHO report on the global tobacco epidemic? 267, 2008.

16. Gilman SL, Zhou X. Smoke. A global history of smoking. University of Chicago Press. 2004.

17. CDC (Centers for Disease Control). The health consequences of smoking: A report of the Surgeon General. www.americanlegacy.org. 2004.

18. Child smoking in father's lap in China outrages world. Daily Telegraph. April 13, 2011.

19. D'Espaingnet ET. WHO report on the global tobacco epidemic, 2013

20. Smoking in Asia: A looming health epidemic. www.asianscientist.com

21. Health at a glance: Asia/Pacific 2012. www.OECD-ilibrary.org

22. World Health Organization. Tobacco Atlas. www.who.int/tobacco/en/atlas.2012

23. Jha P, Ranson MK, Nguyen SN, Yach D. Estimates of Global and Regional Prevalence by age and sex. American Journal of Public Health. 92:1002, 2002.
24. Ginzel KH. What's in a cigarette? www.quitsmokingsupport.com
25. Kleinman L and Messina-Kleinman D. Ingredients in a cigarette. In Smoking, diet and health. www.barnesandandnoble.com
26. Harms of smoking and health benefits of quitting. National Cancer Institute. www.cancer.gov/cancertopics/factsheet/tobacco/cessation.
27. How tobacco smoke causes disease: The Biology and Behavioral Basis for Smoking-Attributable Disease: A report of the Surgeon General. Atlanta. GA. U.S. Department of Health and Human Services. Promotion Office on Smoking and Health, 2004.
28. Djordjevic MV, Doran KA. Nicotine content and delivery across tobacco products. Handbook of Experimental Pharmacology. 192:61, 2009.
29. An Introduction to Indoor Air Quality (IAQ). Carbon Monoxide (CO). www.epa.gov/iaq.co
30. Jha P, Chaloupka FJ, eds. Tobacco control in developing countries. Oxford. England: Oxford University Press. 2000.
31. Murray CJ, Lopez AD. Alternative projections of mortality and disability by cause 1990-2020: Global Burden of Disease Study. Lancet: 349, 1498, 1997.

CHAPTER 2 COUGH

1. Lai K, Luo W, Zeng G, Zhong N. Diagnosis and treatment of chronic cough in China: an insight into the status quo. Cough. 1:21, 2012.
2. Irwin RS, Boulet LP, Cloutier MM, Fuller R, Hoffstein V, Ing AJ, McCool FD, O'Byrne P, Poe RH. Managing cough

as a defense mechanism and as a symptom. Chest. 114:1335, 1998.

3. Chen RC, Lai FK, Liu W, Zhong NS. An epidemiological study of cough in young college students in Guangzhou. Clin J Epidemiol. 27:123, 2006.

4. Kohno S, Ishida T, Uchida Y, Kishimoto H, Sasaki H, Shioya T, Tokuyama K, Niimi A, Nishi K, Fujimura M. The Japanese Respiratory Society Guidelines for management of cough. Respirology. 11; S135, 2006.

5. Woodman L, Sutcliffe A, Kaur D, Berry M, Bradding P, Pavord ID, Brightling CE, Chemokine concentrations and mast cell chemotactic activity in BAL fluid in patients with eosinophilic bronchitis and asthma, and in normal control subjects. Chest. 130:371, 2006.

6. Ziment I. Herbal antitussives. Pulm. Pharmacol. Ther. 15:327, 2002.

7. Chang AB, Glomb WB. Guidelines for evaluating chronic cough in pediatrics: ACCP evidence-based clinical practice guidelines. Chest. 260S, 2006.

8. Lai KF, Li BK, Wang FX, Chen RC, Liu XY, Zhong NS. Survey on the diagnosis and management of the patients with chronic cough. Int J Respir. 31:645, 2011.

9. Morice A. The diagnosis and management of chronic cough. Eur. Respir. J. 24:481, 2004.

10. Society JR. Prolonged and chronic cough. Respirology 11(Suppl):160, 2006.

CHAPTER 3 ASTHMA

WHERE ARE ASTHMA DEATHS OCCURING?

1. Centers for Disease Control and Prevention, National Center for Health Statistics. U.S. report of final mortality statistics, 1979-2001, Atlanta (GA): Centers for Disease Control and Prevention, 2001.

2. National Institutes of Health, National Heart, Lung and Blood Institute. Morbidity and mortality: 2002 chart book on cardiovascular, lung, and blood diseases. Bethesda (MD): U.S. Department of Health and Human Services, Public Health Service, National Institutes of Health; 2002.

3. American Lung Association. Trends in asthma morbidity and mortality. Washington, DC: American Lung Association, Epidemiology and Statistics Unit; 2004.

4. Rebuck AS, The global decline in asthma death rates: can we relax now? Asia Pacific Allergy. 3:1, 2013.

5. International study of Bronchial Asthma and allergies in childhood (ISAAC) world-wide variations in the prevalence of Bronchial Asthma symptoms. European Respir J. 12:315, 1998.

6. World Health Organization. Bronchial Asthma: scope of the problem. www.who.int. 2005.

7. Lai CKW, Kim Y-Y, Kuo S-H, Spencer M, Williams AE, and the Asthma Insights and Reality in Asia Pacific Steering Committee. Cost of Asthma in the Asia-Pacific region. Eur Respir Rev. 15:10, 2006.

8. Pawankar R, Bunnag C, Khaltaev N, Bousquet J. Allergic Rhinitis and Its Impact on Asthma in Asia Pacific and the ARIA Update 2008. World Allergy Organ J. Suppl 3: S212, 2012.

9. Bousquet J, Khaltaev N. Global surveillance, prevention and control of chronic respiratory diseases: a comprehensive approach. Geneva, Switzerland: Global Alliance against Chronic Respiratory Diseases, World Health Organization. 2007.

10. Asher MI, Montefort S, Bjorksten B, Lai CK, Strachan DP, and Weiland SK, Williams H. Worldwide time trends in the prevalence of symptoms of asthma, allergic rhino-conjunctivitis and eczema in childhood: ISAAC Phases One and Three repeat multi-country cross-sectional surveys. Lancet. 368: 733, 2006.

WHY ARE ASTHMA DEATHS OCCURING?

1. Abramson MJ, Bailey MJ, Couper FJ, Driver JS, Drummer OH, Forbes AB, McNeil JJ, Haydn Walters E. Victorian Asthma Mortality Study Group. Are asthma medications and management related to deaths from asthma? Am J Crit Care Med. 163:12, 2001.
2. Kesten S, Rebuck AS. Asthma in New Zealand: implications for North America. J Asthma. 28:193, 1991.
3. Rea HH, Garrett JE, Mulder J, Chapman KR, White JG, Rebuck AS. Emergency room care of asthmatics; a comparison between Auckland and Toronto. Ann Allergy. 66:48, 1991.
4. Horwitz RI, Spitzer W, Buist S, Cockroft D, Boivin JF, McNutt M, Rebuck AS, Suissa S. Clinical complexity and epidemiological uncertainty in case-control research. Fenoterol and asthma management. Chest. 100:1586, 1991.
5. Spitzer WO, Suissa S, Ernst P, Horwitz RI, Habbick B, Cockroft D, Boivin JF, McNutt M, Buist S. Fenoterol and death from asthma. Med J Aust. 157:567, 1992.
6. Spitzer WO, Ernst P, Suissa S, Horwitz RI, Habbick B, Cockroft D, Boivin JF, McNutt M, Buist S, Rebuck AS. The use of beta-agonists and the risk of death and near death from asthma. N Engl J Med. 126:501, 1992.

WHAT CAN BE DONE ABOUT THE INCREASE IN ASTHMA PREVALENCE AND SEVERITY?

1. International study of Bronchial Asthma and allergies in childhood (ISAAC) world-wide variations in the prevalence of Bronchial Asthma symptoms. European Respir J. 12:315, 1998.
2. http://isaac.auckland.ac.nz/publications/publicationsintro.html
3. Partridge MR. Has ISAAC told us as much as it can? Where now? Thorax. 64:462, 2009.

4. Enarson DA. Fostering a spirit of critical thinking: the ISAAC story. Int J Tuberc Lung Dis. 9:1,2005.
5. World Health Organization. Global alliance against chronic respiratory disease (GARD) basket: a package of information, surveillance tools and guidelines to be offered as a service to countries. Geneva. World Health Organization; 2008.
6. Gakidou E, Oza S, Fuertes CV, Lee DK, Soussa A, Hogan MC. et al. Improving child survival through environmental and nutritional interventions: the importance of targeting interventions toward the poor. JAMA. 298:1876, 2007.

TREATMENT GUIDELINES

1. Bousquet J, Clark TJH, Hurd S, Khaltaev N, Lenfant C, O'Byrne P, Sheffer A. GINA guidelines on asthma and beyond. Allergy. 62:102, 2007.
2. Jackson R, Feder G. Guidelines for clinical guidelines. BMJ. 317:427, 1998.
3. Global strategy for asthma management and prevention. WHO/NHLBI workshop report. Lung and Blood Institute: National Institutes of Health, National Heart, Publication Number95-3659, 1995.
4. http://www.ginasthma.com
5. Cabana MD, Rand CS, Becher OJ, Rubin HR. Reasons for pediatrician non-adherence to asthma guidelines. Arch Pediatr Adolesc Med. 155:1057, 2001.
6. Bateman ED, Boushey HA, Bousquet J, Busse WW, Clark TJ, Pauwels RA et al. Can guideline-defined asthma control be achieved? The Gaining Optimal Asthma Control Study. Am J Crit Care Med. 170:836, 2004.
7. Masoli M, Fabian D, Holt S, Beasley R. The global burden of asthma: executive summary of the GINA Dissemination Committee Report. Allergy. 59:469, 2004.

8. Chapman KR, Ernst P, Grenville A, Dewland P, Zimmerman S. Control of Asthma in Canada: failure to achieve guideline targets. Can Respir J. 8(Suppl):35, 2001.

9. Brown R, Bratton SL, Cabana MD, Kaciroti N, Clark NM. Physician asthma education program improves outcomes for children of low-income families. Chest 126:369, 2004.

10. Morishima T, Otsubo T, Gotou E, Kobayashi D, Lee J, Imanaka Y. Physician adherence to asthma treatment guidelines in Japan: focus on inhaled corticosteroids. Journal of Evaluation in Clinical Practice. 19:223, 2013.

11. Cabana MD, Slish KK, Evans D, Mellins RB, Brown RW, Lin X, Kaciroti N, Clark NM. Impact of Physician Asthma Care Education on Patient Outcomes. Pediatrics. 117:2149, 2006.

12. Lai CKW, de Guia T, Lloyd A, Williams AE, Spencer MD. Asthma control and its direct healthcare costs: findings using a derived Asthma Control Test score in eight Asia-Pacific areas. European Respiratory Review. 15:24, 2006.

13. Fang X, Li S, Gao L, Zhao N, Wang X, Bai C. A short-term education program improved physicians' adherence for COPD and asthma in Shanghai. Clin Transl Med. 1:13, 2013.

14. Kang M-K, Kim B-K, Kim T-W, Kim S-H, Kang H-R, Park H-W, Chang Y-S, Kim S-S, Min K-U, Kim Y-Y, Cho S-H. Physicians' Preference for Asthma Guidelines Implementation. Allergy Asthma Immunol Res. 2:247, 2010.

15. Patel MR, Shah S, Cabana MD, Sawyer SM, Toelle B, Mellis C, Jenkins C, Brown RW, Clark N. Translation of an evidence-based asthma intervention: Physician Asthma Care Education (PACE) in the United States and Australia. Primary Care Respiratory Journal. 22:29, 2013.

CHAPTER 4 COPD

What is it and why is it so difficult to understand?
Definition, size of the problem, physiology and causes:

1. ERS Respiratory Roadmap. Recommendations for the future of respiratory medicine, Health Policy Makers version, Research Chapter, published June 2011.
2. Murray CJL, Lopez AD. The global burden of disease: a comprehensive assessment of mortality and disability from diseases, injury and risk factors in 1990 and projected to 2020. Cambridge, MA: Harvard University Press, 1996.
3. Lopez AD, Shibuya K, Rao C, et al. Chronic obstructive pulmonary disease: current burden and future projections. Eur Respir J. 27:397, 2006.
4. US Department of Health and Human Services, 2003.
5. Calverley PMA and Walker P. Chronic obstructive pulmonary disease. Lancet, 362: 1053, 2003.
6. Chang-Yeung M, Ait-Khaled N, White N, Ip MS, and Tan WC. The burden of COPD in Asia and Africa. Int J Tuberc Lung Dis. 8:12, 2004.
7. Fishman AP. One hundred years of chronic obstructive pulmonary disease. Am J Respir Crit Care Med. 171:941, 2005.
8. Shim YS. Epidemiological survey of chronic obstructive pulmonary disease and alpha-1 antitrypsin deficiency in Korea. Respirology. 6 (Suppl):S9, 2001.
9. Prevalence of COPD in Europe according to the Organization for Economic Co-operation and Development. www.oecd.org
10. Petty TL. The history of COPD. Int J Chronic Obstruct Pulm Dis. 1:3, 2006.
11. Buist S, et al. Expanding our knowledge of COPD. Lancet. 370:733, 2007.
12. Buist AS, McBurnie MA, Vollmer WM, Gillespie S, Burney P, Mannino DM, Menezes AM, Sullivan SD,

Lee TA, Weiss KB, Jensen RL, Marks GB, Gulsvik A, Nizankowska-Mogilnicka E. BOLD Collaborative Research Group. International variation in the prevalence of COPD (the BOLD Study): a population-based prevalence study. Lancet. 370:741, 2007.

13. Global Initiative for Chronic Obstructive Lung Disease. Global strategy for the diagnosis, management, and prevention of chronic obstructive pulmonary disease. NIH, NHLBI 2701. Bathesda, MD: NHLBI/WHO report, April, 2001.

14. Fletcher C, Petro R. The natural history of chronic airflow obstruction. BMJ. 1:1645, 1977.

15. Calverley PM, Koulouris NG. Flow limitation and dynamic hyperinflation: key concepts in modern respiratory physiology. Eur Resp J. 25:186,2005.

16. Hogg JC, Chu F, Utokaparch S, et al. The nature of small airway obstruction in chronic obstructive pulmonary disease. N Engl J Med. 350:2645, 2004.

17. O'Donnell DE. Hyperinflation, Dyspnea and Exercise Intolerance in Chronic Obstructive Pulmonary Disease. The Proceedings of the American Thoracic Society. 3:180, 2006.

18. Bates DV. The fate of chronic bronchitis: a report of the ten-year follow-up in the Canadian Veterans Affairs Coordinated study of chronic bronchitis. Am Rev Respir Dis. 108:1043, 1973?

19. World Health Organization. Smoking Prevalence. In: Tobacco or Health: A Global Status Report. Geneva, Switzerland: WHO, pp 10-18, 1979.

20. Salvi SS, Manap R, Beasley R. Understanding the true burden of COPD: the epidemiological challenges. Prim Care Respir J. 21, 2012.

21. Anthonisen NR, Connett JE, Murray RP. Smoking and lung function of Lung Health Study Participants after 11 years. Am J Crit Care Med. 166:675, 2002.

22. Mannino DM. Chronic obstructive pulmonary disease: definition and epidemiology. Respir Care. 48:1185, 2003.
23. Buist AS, Bailey W, Hurd SS. National COPD Conference Summary. J COPD. 1:293,2000.
24. www.nlm.nih.gov/medlineplus/ *copd*chronicobstructivepulmonarydisease
25. physicsdaily.com/physics/Lung
26. Physics: Principles with Applications (5th Edition) by Douglas C. Giancoli, Hardcover: 1096 pages, Publisher: Prentice Hall
27. Principles of Physics (with PhysicsNow and InfoTrac) by Raymond A. Serway, John W. Jewett, Hardcover: 1320 pages, Publisher: Brooks Cole.
28. Schaum's Outline of College Physics by Frederick J. Bueche, Eugene Hecht, Paperback: 416 pages, Publisher: McGraw-Hill

CHAPTER 5 IS COPD FATAL?

1. www.netterimages.com/artist/netter
2. Petty TL. COPD Clinical Phenotypes. Pulm Pharmacol Ther. 15:341, 2002.
3. Johnson MA, Woodcock AA, Rehahn M and Geddes DM. Are 'pink puffers' more breathless than 'blue bloaters'? BMJ (Clinical Research Ed.).286:179, 1983.
4. International COPD Coalition. Quick facts about COPD. www.internationalcopd.org/materials/patients.
5. Stockley RA, Mannino D, Barnes PJ. Burden and pathogenesis of chronic obstructive pulmonary disease. Proc Am Thorac Soc. 6:524, 2009.
6. Hansell AL, Walk JA, Soriano JB. What do patients with chronic obstructive pulmonary disease die from? A multiple cause coding analysis. Eur Respir J. 22:809, 2003.
7. Zielinski J, MacNee W, Wedzicha J, Ambrosino N, Braghiroli A, Dolensky J, Howard P, Gorzelak K,

Lahdensuo A, Strom K, Tobiasz M and Weitzenblum E. Causes of death in patients with COPD and chronic respiratory failure. Monaldi Arch Chest Dis 52:43, 1997.

8. Restrepo MI, Mortensen EM, Pugh JA and Anzueto A. COPD is associated with increased mortality in patients with community-acquired pneumonia. European Respiratory Journal. 28:346, 2006.

9. Chapman KR, Mannino DM, Soriano JB et al. Epidemiology and costs of chronic obstructive pulmonary disease. Eur Respir J. 27:188, 2006.

10. Jensen HH, Godffredsen NS, Lange P, et al. Potential misclassification of causes of death from COPD. Eur Respir J. 28:781, 2006.

11. Celli BR. Update on the management of COPD. Chest.133: 1451, 2008

12. Rennard SI. COPD: overview of definitions, epidemiology, and factors influencing its development. Chest;113(Suppl 4):235,1998.

13. Brown DW, Croft JB, Greenlund KJ, WH Giles WH. Deaths from Chronic Obstructive Pulmonary Disease— United States, 2000-2005. *Div of Adult and Community Health, National Center for Chronic Disease Prevention and Health Promotion, CDC.* MMWR. 57(45); 1229, 2008.

14. Soriano Ortiz JB, Almagro P, Sauleda Roig J. Causes of mortality in COPD. Arch Bronconeumol. 45 Suppl 4:8,2009.

CHAPTER 6 HOW COMMON IS COPD IN ASIA?

1. Rebuck AS. COPD in Asia is a gathering storm. Biospectrum. 13 June, 2013.

2. Murray C J L, Lopez A D. The global burden of disease: a comprehensive assessment of mortality and disability from

diseases, injury and risk factors in 1990 and projected to 2020. Cambridge, MA: Harvard University Press, 1996.

3. Lopez A D, Shibuya K, Rao C, et al. Chronic obstructive pulmonary disease: current burden and future projections. Eur Respir J. 27:397-412, 2006.

4. US Department of Health and Human Services, 2003.

5. Calverley P M A and Walker P. Chronic obstructive pulmonary disease. Lancet, 362: 1053-61, 2003.

6. Chang-Yeung M, Ait-Khaled N, White N, Ip M S and Tan WC. The burden and impact of COPD in Asia and Africa. Int J Tuberc Lung Dis. 8:12-14, 2004.

7. Regional COPD Working Group. COPD prevalence in 12 Asia-Pacific countries and regions: projections based on the COPD prevalence model. Respirology. 8:192-8, 2003.

8. Shim Y S. Epidemiological survey of chronic obstructive pulmonary disease and alpha-1 antitrypsin deficiency in Korea. Respirology. 6 (Suppl): S9-S11, 2001

9. Izumi T. Chronic obstructive lung disease in Japan. Curr Opin Pulm Med. 8:102-105, 2002.

10. Buist AS, McBurnie MA, Vollmer WM, Gillespie S, Burney P, Mannino DM, Menezes AM, Sullivan SD, Lee TA, Weiss KB, Jensen RL, Marks GB, Gulsvik A, Nizankowska-Mogilnicka E; BOLD Collaborative Research Group. International variation in the prevalence of COPD (the BOLD Study): a population-based prevalence study. Lancet.370:741, 2007.

11. Global Initiative for Chronic Obstructive Lung Disease. Global strategy for the diagnosis, management, and prevention of chronic obstructive pulmonary disease. NIH, NHLBI 2701. Bathesda, MD: NHLBI/WHO report, April, 2001.

12. Fletcher C, Petro R. The natural history of chronic airflow obstruction. BMJ. 1:1645-1648, 1977.

13. Bates D V. The fate of chronic bronchitis: a report of the ten-year follow-up in the Canadian Veterans Affairs

Coordinated study of chronic bronchitis. Am Rev Respir Dis. 108:1043-1065, 1973.

14. World Health Organization. Smoking Prevalence. In: Tobacco or Health: A Global Status Report. Geneva, Switzerland: World Health Organization, pp 10-18, 1997.

15. Drummond MB, Dasenbrook EC, Pitz MW, Murphy DJ, Fan E. Inhaled corticosteroids in patients with stable chronic obstructive pulmonary disease: a systemic review and meta-analysis. JAMA. 300:2407-16, 2008.

16. Tan WC. The global initiative for chronic obstructive lung disease: Gold standards and the Asia-Pacific perspective. Respirology.7:1-2, 2002.

17. Pawels RA, Buist SA, Calverley PMA, Jenkins CR, Hurd S. Global strategy for the diagnosis, management and prevention of chronic obstructive pulmonary disease. Am J Respir Crit Care Med. 163: 1256-1276, 2001.

18. Tan WC, Ng TP. COPD in Asia: where East meets West. Chest.133:517-27, 2008.

19. Jindal SK. COPD: The unrecognized epidemic in India. Suppl. To JAPI. 60:14, 2012.

CHAPTER 7 MANAGEMENT OF COPD

Smoking cessation, oxygen, surgery and rehabilitation.

1. Fletcher C, Peto R, Tinker C, Speizer FE. The natural history of chronic bronchitis and emphysema. London: Oxford University Press. 1976.

2. Rebuck AS, Vandenberg RA: The relationship between pulmonary artery pressure and physiological dead space in obstructive lung disease. Am Rev Respir Dis 107:423,1973.

3. Rebuck AS. Current Therapy in Respiratory Disease (R.M.Cherniack; publ. B.C. Dekker) "Acute Respiratory Failure in Chronic Obstructive Pulmonary Disease."

4. Rebuck AS. Chronic Obstructive Pulmonary Disease. (N.S Cherniack) Publ. W.B. Saunders. "Respiratory Stimulants in the Treatment of COPD."

5. Rebuck AS, Chapman KR, Abboud R, Pare PD, Kreisman H, Wolkove N, D'Urzo AD, Vickerson F: Nebulized anticholinergic and sympathomimetic treatment of asthma and chronic obstructive airways disease in the emergency room. Am J Med 82:59-64, 1987.

6. Kesten S, Rebuck AS: Management of chronic obstructive pulmonary disease. Drugs 38:160-174, 1989.

7. Croxton TL, Weinmann GG, Senior RM and Hoidal JR. Future Research Directions in Chronic Obstructive Pulmonary Disease. Am J Respir Crit Care Med. 165:838, 2002.

8. How tobacco smoke Causes Disease: The Biology and Behavioral Basis for Smoking-Attributable Disease. U.S.Department of Health and Human Services.: A Report of the Surgeon General, Atlanta, GA:U.S. Department of Health and Human Services, Centers for Disease Control and Prevention, National Center for Chronic Disease Prevention and Health Promotion, Office on Smoking and Health, 2010.

9. The Health Benefits of Smoking Cessation. U.S. Department of Health and Human Services. Rockville, MD. Office on Smoking and Health. 1990.

10. Anthonisen NR, Connett JE, Kiley JP et al. Effects of smoking intervention and the use of an inhaled anti-cholinergic bronchodilator on the rate of decline of FEV_1. JAMA. 272:1497, 1994.

11. West R and Shiffman S. Fast Facts: Smoking Cessation. Health Press Ltd. P. 28, 2007.

12. Anthonisen NR, Skeans MA, Wise RA, et al. Effects of smoking intervention on 14.5 year mortality: a randomized clinical trial. Ann Intern Med. 142:233, 2005.

13. Rabe KF, Hurd H, Anzueto A et al. Global Strategy for the Diagnosis, Management and Prevention of Chronic

Obstructive Pulmonary Disease: GOLD Executive Summary. Am J Crit Care Med. 176:532,2007.

14. Fletcher C, Petro R. The natural history of chronic airflow obstruction. BMJ. 1:1645, 1977.

15. Stoller JK, Panos RJ, Krachman S, Doherty DE, Make B, and the Long-term Oxygen Treatment Trial Research Group. Chest. 138:179. 2010.

16. Croxton TL, Bailey WC. Long-term oxygen treatment in chronic obstructive pulmonary disease: recommendations for future research: an NHLBI workshop report. Am J Respir Crit Care Med. 174:373, 2006.

17. Doherty DE, Petty TL, Bailey W, et al. Recommendations of the 6th long-term oxygen therapy consensus conference. Respir Care.51: 519, 2006.

18. Report of the Medical Research Council Working Party Long term domiciliary oxygen therapy in chronic hypoxic cor pulmonale complicating chronic bronchitis and emphysema. Lancet. 1:681,1981.

19. Nocturnal Oxygen Therapy Trial Group Continuous or nocturnal oxygen therapy in hypoxemic chronic obstructive lung disease: a clinical trial. Ann Intern Med. 93:391,1980.

20. Weitzenblum E, Sautegeau A, Ehrhart M, Mammosser M, Pelletier A. Long-term oxygen therapy can reverse the progression of pulmonary hypertension in patients with chronic obstructive pulmonary disease. Am Rev Respir Dis. 131:493,1985.

21. Cranston JM, Crockett AJ, Moss JR, Alpers JH. Domiciliary oxygen for chronic obstructive pulmonary disease. Cochrane Database Syst Rev. 2005.

22. Bergofsky EH. Tissue oxygen delivery and cor pulmonale in chronic obstructive pulmonary disease. N Engl J Med. 308:1092, 1983.

23. Gorecka D, Gorzelak K, Sliwinski P, et al. Effect of long-term oxygen therapy on survival in patients with chronic obstructive pulmonary disease with moderate hypoxemia. Thorax. 52:674, 1997.

24. Fishman A, Martinez F, Naunheim K, et al. A randomized trial comparing lung-volume-reduction surgery with medical therapy for severe emphysema. N Engl J Med. 348:2059, 2003.

25. Hopkins PM, Seale H, Walsh J, Tam R, Kermeen F, Bell S and McNeil K. Long-term results post conventional lung volume reduction surgery exceeds outcome of lung transplantation for emphysema. Journal of Heart and Lung Transplantation. 25:S61, 2005.

26. COPD. Treatments and drugs. www.mayoclinic.com/health/copd

27. www.lung.ca/diseases-maladies/copd-mpoc/treatment

28. Lung reduction surgery. www.siumed.edu/news

29. Lacasse Y, Brosseau L, Milne S et al. "Pulmonary rehabilitation for chronic obstructive pulmonary disease". In Lacasse, Yves. *Cochrane database of systematic reviews* (2002).

30. Ferreira IM, Brooks D, White J, Goldstein R. "Nutritional supplementation for stable chronic obstructive pulmonary disease". *Cochrane Database Syst Rev* **12,** 2012.

31. Puhan MA, Gimeno-Santos E, Scharplatz M, Troosters T, Walters EH, Steurer J "Pulmonary rehabilitation following exacerbations of chronic obstructive pulmonary disease". *Cochrane Database Syst Rev* (10), 2011.

32. Goldstein RS, Gort EH, Avendano MA, Guyatt GH. Randomized controlled trial of respiratory rehabilitation. The Lancet. 344:1394, 1994.

33. Nici L, Donner C, Wouters E, et al. American Thoracic Society/European Respiratory Society statement on pulmonary rehabilitation. Amer J Resp Crit Care. 173:1390,2006.

34. Santus P, Bassi L, Radovanovic D, Airoldi A, Raccanelli R, Triscan F, Giovannelli F and Spanevello A. Pulmonary Rehabilitation in COPD: A reappraisal (2008-2012). Pulm Med. 10:1155, 2013.

35. Ahmedzai S, Balfour-Lynn IM, Bewick T et al. Managing passengers with stable respiratory disease planning air travel:

British Thoracic Society recommendations. Thorax 2011; 66 Suppl 1, 2011.

CHAPTER 8 TREATMENT OF COPD

Pharmacological therapy

1. http://www.nhlbi.nih.gov/health/health-topics/topics/copd
2. http://copd.about.com/od/copdtreatment/tp/Copd-Treatment-Guidelines.htm
3. *Global Strategy for the Diagnosis, Management and Prevention of COPD*, Global Initiative for Chronic Obstructive Lung Disease (GOLD) 2013. http://www.goldcopd.org/.
4. Abbatecola AM, Fumagalli A, Bonardi D, Guffanti EE. Practical management problems of chronic obstructive pulmonary disease in the elderly: acute exacerbations. Curr Opin Pulm Med.17 Suppl 1:S49, 2011.
5. Chapman KR, Rennard SI, Dogra A, Owen R, Lassen C, Kramer B. Long-term safety and efficacy of indacaterol, a long-acting beta(2)-agonist, in subjects with COPD: a randomized, placebo-controlled study. Chest.140: 68, 2011.
6. Chong J, Karner C, Poole P. Tiotropium versus long-acting beta-agonists for stable chronic obstructive pulmonary disease. Cochrane Database Syst Rev, 107, 2012.
7. Lee SD, Hui DS, Mahayiddin AA, et al. Roflumilast in Asian patients with COPD: A randomized placebo-controlled trial. Respirology.16: 1249, 2011.
8. Mahler DA, D'Urzo A, Bateman ED, et al. Concurrent use of indacaterol plus tiotropium in patients with COPD provides superior bronchodilation compared with tiotropium alone: a randomized, double-blind comparison. Thorax; 67:781, 2012.
9. Tashkin DP, Doherty DE, Kerwin E, et al. Efficacy and safety of a fixed-dose combination of mometasone furoate

and formoterol fumarate in subjects with moderate to very severe COPD: results from a 52-week Phase III trial. Int J Chron Obstruct Pulmon Dis; 7:43, 2012.

10. https://www.icsi.org/guidelines FDA approves GSK/ Theravance COPD drug Breo Ellipta. World News. May 13, 2013.Tan WC, Ng TPCOPD in Asia: where East meets West. Chest.133(2): 517, 2008.

11. Global Initiative for Chronic Obstructive Lung Disease strategy for the diagnosis, management and prevention of chronic obstructive pulmonary disease: An Asia-Pacific perspective. THE ASIA PACIFIC COPD ROUNDTABLE GROUP. Respirology 1:9; 2005.

CHAPTER 9 COPD RESEARCH

Drugs in the pipeline.

1. Barnes PJ. Development of new drugs for COPD. Curr Med Chem. 20:1531, 2013.

2. Mercardo N, Thimmulappa R, Thomas CMR, Fenwick PS, Chana KK, Donnelly LE, Biswal S, Ito K, and Barnes PJ. Decreased histone deacetylase 2 impairs Nrf2 activation by oxidative stress. Biochem Biophys Res Commun. 406:292, 2011.

3. Boutten A, Goven D, Artaud-Macari E, Boczkowski J, Bonay M. NRF2 targeting: a promising therapeutic strategy in chronic obstructive pulmonary disease.Trends Mol Med. 17:363, 2011.

4. Boutten A, Goven D, Aartaud-Macari E, Bonay M. Protective role of Nrf2 in the lungs against oxidative airway disease. Med Sci (Paris). 27:966, 2011.

5. Cho HY and Kleeberger SR. Nrf2 protects against airway disorders. Toxicol Appl Pharmacol. 244:43, 2010.

6. What is a histone deacetylase inhibitor? www.askives.com.

7. Kazuhiro I, Ito M, Elliott M, Cosio B, Caramori G, Kon OM, Barczyk A, Hayashi S, Adcock IM, Hogg JC and Barnes PJ.Decreased Histone Deacetylase Activity in Chronic Obstructive Pulmonary Disease. N Engl J Med. 352:1967, 2005.
8. Chung KF. P38 mitogen-activated protein kinase pathways in asthma and COPD. Chest. 139:1470, 2011.
9. Gaffey K, Reynolds S, Plumb J, Kaur M and Singh D. Increased phosphorylated p38 mitogen-activated protein kinase in COPD lungs. Eur Resp J. 42:28, 2013.
10. Renda T, Baraldo S, Pelaia G, Bazzan E. Turato G, Papi A, Maestrelli P, Maselli R, Vatrella A, Fabbri LM, Zuin R, Marsico SA and saetta M. Increased activation of p38 MAPK in COPD. Eur Respir J. 1:62, 2008.
11. Ratcliffe MJ and Dougall MJ. Comparison of the anti-inflammatory effects of Cilomast, Budesonide and a p38 Mitogen activated protein kinase inhibitor in COPD lung tissue macrophages. BMC Pharmacology and Toxicology. 13:15, 2012.

CHAPTER 10 COPD: ACTION PLANS

Surely there is more we can do.

1. http://www.copdcoalition.eu/what_we_do/call-to-action
2. http://www.aarc.org/headlines/13/04/copd_research.cfm
3. http://www.internationalcopd.org/documents/English/ CallToAction.
4. The European COPD Coalition calls for action to be taken at the European, national and local levels to tackle the epidemic of COPD. http://www.copdcoalition.eu/ ECC-Call-to-Action-on-COPD.
5. Peter D. Wagner, President, ATS. Sonia Buist, Past President, ATS Richard Casaburi, Co-Chair, ATS Pulmonary Rehabilitation Section and

Bartolome Celli. http://www.newswise.com/articles/
lung-experts-for-copd-day

6. Goldstein RS. http://www.lung.ca/_resources/
Women_COPD_Presentation_2006.

7. COPD Research Funding. http://research.copdfoundation.
org/funding_sources

CHAPTER 11 LUNG FUNCTION TESTING IN COPD

Is the FEV$_1$ outdated?

1. History of the Boston University Pulmonary Section.www.
bumc.bu.edu/pulmonary/pastandpresent/history.

2. Lung function testing: selection of reference values and
interpretive strategies. Am Rev Respir Dis. 144:1202, 1991.

3. Hankinson JL, Odencranz JR, Fedan KB. Spirometric
reference values from a sample of the general US
population. Am Rev Respir Crit Care Med. 159:179, 1999.

4. Swanney MP, Beckert LE, Frampton CM et al. Validity
of the American Thoracic Society and other spirometric
algorithms using FVC and Forced Expiratory Volume at
6s for predicting a reduced Total Lung Capacity. Chest.
126:1861,2004.

5. Kesten S and Rebuck AS. Is the short-term response to
inhaled beta-adrenergic agonist sensitive or specific for
distinguishing between Asthma and COPD? Chest.
105:1042, 1994.

6. Gelb AF, Gutierrez A, Weisman IM et al. Simplified
Detection of Dynamic Hyperinflation. Chest. 126: 1855,
2004.

7. Celli BR, MacNee W et al. Standards for the diagnosis and
treatment of patients with COPD: a summary of the ATS/
ERS position paper. Eur Respir J. 23:932, 2004.

8. Taube C, Lehnigk B, Paasch K et al. Factor analysis of
changes in dyspnea and lung volume parameters in chronic

obstructive pulmonary disease. Am J Respir Crit Care Med. 162: 216, 2000.

9. Woolcock AJ, Rebuck AS, Cade JF, Read JR. Lung volume changes in asthma measured concurrently by two methods. Am Rev Respir Dis. 104:73, 1071.

10. Rodarte JR, Noredin G, Miller C et al. Lung elastic recoil during breathing at increased lung volume. J Appl Physiol. 87:1491, 1999.

11. Waterhouse JC, Pritchard SM, Howard P. Hyperinflation, trapped gas and theophylline in chronic obstructive pulmonary disease. Monaldi Arch Chest Dis. 48:126, 1993.

12. Duranti R, Filippelli M, Bianchi R, Romagnili I et al. Inspiratory capacity and decrease in lung hyperinflation with Albuterol in COPD. Chest. 122: 2009, 2002.

13. Suissa S. Lung function decline in COPD trials: bias from regression to the mean. Eur Respir J. 32:829, 2008.

14. Richard Johnston. Observations, opinions and ideas about pulmonary function testing. FEV_6. www.pftforum.com/blog/FEV_6

15. Jones P, Miravitlles M, van der Molen T and Kulich K. Beyond FEV_1 in COPD: a review of patient-reported outcomes and their measurement. Int J Chron Obstructive Pulmon Dis. 7:697, 2012.

16. Borrill ZL, Houghton CM, Woodcock AA and Singh D. Measuring bonchodilation in COPD clinical trials. Br J Pharmacol. 59:379, 2005.

17. Kesten S, Celli B, Decramer M, Liu D and Tashkin D. Adverse health consequences in COPD patients with rapid decline in FEV_1—evidence from the UPLIFT trial. Respir Res. 12: 129, 2011.

18. Perez-Padilla R, Wehrmeister FC, Celli BR, Lopez-Varela MV, de Oca MM, Muino A, Talamo C, Jardim JR, Valdivia G, Lisboa C, Menezes AMB and the PLATINO Team. Reliability of FEV_1/FEV_6 to diagnose airflow obstruction compared with FEV_1/FVC: The PLATINO Longitudinal Study. PLoS One. 8:2013.

19. Vestbo J, Anderson W, Coxson HO, Crim C, Dawber F, Edwards L, Hagan G, Knobil K, Lomas DA, MacNee W, Silverman EK, Tal-Singer R and on behalf of the ECLIPSE investigators. Eur Resp J. 4:869, 2008.

20. Aboussouan LS and Stoller JK. Flow-volume loops. Overview of pulmonary function testing in adults. www. uptodate.com/contents/flow-volume—loops.

21. Akkermans RP, Berrevoets MA, Smeele IJ, Lucas AE, Thoonen BP, Grootens-Stekelenburg JG, Heijdra YF, van Weel C and Schermer TR. Lung function decline in relation to diagnostic criteria for airflow obstruction in respiratory symptomatic subjects. BMC Pulmonary Medicine. 12:12, 2012.

EPILOGUE COPD and DIABETES

Time bombs and gathering storms

1. Cooper ME and Rebuck AS. Type 2 Diabetes in Asia: A threat to human health and well-being—J of Diabetes 2013 Oct 17. doi: 10.1111/1753-0407.12097.

2. International Diabetes Federation. IDF Diabetes Atlas. Brussels: International Diabetes Federation, 2011.

3. Whiting DR, Guariguata L, Weil C, Shaw J. IDF Atlas: global estimates of the prevalence of the prevalence of diabetes for 2011 and 2030. Diabetes research and clinical practice. 94:311, 2011.

4. Chen L, Magliano DJ, Zimmet PZ. The worldwide epidemic of type 2 diabetes mellitus—present and future perspectives. Nature reviews Endocrinology. 8:228, 2012.

5. Gluckman PD, Hanson MA, Cooper C. Effects of in utero and early-life conditions on adult and health and disease. The New England Journal of Medicine. 359:61, 2008.

6. Global Initiative for Chronic Obstructive Lung Disease. Global strategy for the diagnosis, management and

prevention of chronic obstructive lung disease. NIH, NHLBI 2701. Bethesda, MD: NHLBI/WHO report, April, 2011.

7. Soriano JB, Lamprecht B. Chronic Obstructive Pulmonary Disease: A worldwide problem. Med Clin N Am. 96:671, 2012.

8. Chang-Yeung M, Ait-Kahlid N, White N et al. The burden and impact of COPD in Asia and Africa. Int J Tuberc Lung Dis. 8:12, 2004.

9. Rebuck AS. COPD in Asia is a gathering storm. Biospectrum. 13 June, 2013.

10. Shaw JE, Sicree RA, Zimmet PZ. Global estimates of the prevalence of diabetes for 2010 and 2030. Diabetes research and clinical practice. 87:4,2010.

11. Ulvi OS, Chaudhary RY, Ali T, *et al.* investigating the awareness level about Diabetes Mellitus and associated factors in Tarlai (Rural Islamabad). Journal of Pakistan Medical Association. November, 2009.

12. Sabri AS, Qayyum MA, Saigol NU *et al.* Comparing knowledge of diabetes mellitus among rural and urban diabetics. McGill J Med. 10:87, 2007.

13. Yun LS, Hassan Y, Aziz NA, Aaisu A, Ghazali R. A comparison of knowledge of diabetes mellitus between patients with diabetes and healthy adults: a survey from north Malaysia. Patient Educ Couns. 69:47,2007.

14. Halimic A, Gage H, Vrikki M, Williams P. Diabetes awareness and Behavioral Risk Factors among University Students in Saudi Arabia. Middle East Journal of Family Medicine. 11:4,2013.

15. Magliano JD, Soderberg S, Zimmet PZ et al. Explaining the Increase of Diabetes Prevalence and Plasma Glucose in Mauritius. Diabetes Care. 35: 87, 2012.

16. Xu S, Ming J, Gao B, et al. Regional differences in diabetes prevalence and awareness between coastal and interior provinces in China: a population-based cross-over sectional study. BMC Public Health. 13:299,2013.

17. McNeely MJ and Boyko EJ. Type 2 Diabetes Prevalence in Asian Americans: Results of a national health survey. Diabetes Care. 27:66, 2004.
18. Anjana M, Sandeep S, Deepa R et al. Visceral and central abdominal fat in relation to diabetes in Asian Indians. Diabetes Care. 12:2948, 2004.
19. Staimez LR, Weber MB, Ranjani H, et al. Evidence of Reduced Beta Cell Function in Asian Indians With Mild Dysglycemia. Diabetes Care (in press).
20. Gregg EW, Chen H, Wagenknecht LE, et al. Association of an intensive lifestyle intervention with remission of type 2 diabetes. JAMA. 308:2489,2012.
21. Global Initiative for Chronic Obstructive Lung Disease. Global strategy for the diagnosis, management, and prevention of chronic obstructive pulmonary disease. NIH, NHLBI 2701. Bathesda, MD: NHLBI/WHO report, April, 2001.
22. National Report Card on Chronic Obstructive Pulmonary Disease. Canadian Lung Association and Canadian Thoracic Society. http://www.copdcanada.ca/nationally.htm
23. Murray CJL and Lopez AD. The Global Burden of Disease: a comprehensive assessment of mortality and disability from diseases, injury and risk factors in 1090 and projected to 2020. Cambridge, MA: Harvard University Press, 1996.
24. Fuller JH, Elford J, Goldblatt P, Adelstein AM. Diabetes mortality: new light on an underestimated public health problem. Diabetologia. 24:336, 1983.
25. US Department of Health and Human Services, 2002.
26. Hu FB. Globalization of Diabetes: the role of diet, lifestyle and genes. Diabetes Care. 34:1249, 2011.
27. DeFronzo RA, Abdul-Ghani M. Type 2 diabetes can be prevented with early pharmacological intervention. Diabetes Care. 34. Suppl.2:S202, 2011.
28. Kahn SE, Hafner SM, Heise MA et al. Glycemic durability of rosiglitazone, metformin, or glyburide monotherapy. New England Journal of Medicine. 355:2427,2006.

29. Wilson E. Wardle EV, Chandel P, Walford S. Diabetes Education: an Asian perspective. Diabetic Medicine: a journal of the British Diabetic Association. 10:177,1993.
30. Li G, Zhang P, Wang J et al. The long-term effect of lifestyle interventions to prevent diabetes in the China Da Qing Diabetes Prevention Study: a 20-year follow-up study. Lancet 371:1783, 2008.
31. Tuomilehto J, Lindstrom J, Erriksson JG et al. Finnish Diabetes Prevention Study. Prevention of type 2 diabetes mellitus by changes in lifestyle among subjects with impaired glucose tolerance. The New England Journal of Medicine. 244:1343, 2001.
32. Knowler WC, Barrett-Connor E, Fowler SE et al. Diabetes Prevention Program Research. Reduction in the incidence of type 2 diabetes with lifestyle intervention or metformin. The New England Journal of Medicine. 346:393, 2002.
33. Buist AS et al. Expanding our knowledge of COPD. Lancet. 370:733, 2007.
34. Asian Tribune. Diabetes leadership forum seeks solutions to reduce long-term public healthcare costs. Sunday November 1, 2009.
35. US Department of Health and Human Services, 2003.
36. Majikela-Dlangamandla B, Isiavwe A, Levitt N. Diabetes Monitoring in Developing Countries. Diabetes Voice. 51:28, 2006.
37. Danaei G, Finucane MM, Lu Y et al. Global Burden of Metabolic Risk Factors of Chronic Diseases Collaborating. National, regional, and global trends in fasting plasma glucose and diabetes prevalence since 1980: systematic analysis of health examination surveys and epidemiological studies with 370 country-years and 2.7 million participants. Lancet, 378:31, 2011.
38. Di Marco R, Accordini S, Cerveri I et al. Incidence of Chronic Obstructive Pulmonary Disease in a Cohort of Young Adults According to the Presence of Chronic Cough

and Phlegm. American Journal of Respiratory and Critical Care Medicine. 175:32, 2007.

39. Kaufman FR. Type 2 diabetes mellitus in children and youth: a new epidemic. Journal of Pediatric Endocrinology and Metabolism. JPEM 15: Suppl 2:737, 2002.
40. Shim YS. Epidemiological survey of chronic obstructive pulmonary disease and alpha-1 antitrypsin deficiency in Korea. Respirology. 6(Suppl):S9, 2001.
41. DeFronzo RA. Banting Lecture. From the triumvirate to the ominous octet: a new paradigm for the treatment of type 2 diabetes mellitus. Diabetes. 58:773, 2009.
42. Burdge GC and Lillicrop KA. Nutrition, epigenetics, and development plasticity: implications for understanding human disease. Annual review of nutrition. 30:315, 2010.